# ASHP's **Clinical PEARLS**

## Bruce Canaday, PharmD

Clinical Professor and Vice-Chair
Division of Pharmacy Practice and
  Experiential Education
University of North Carolina,
  Eshelman School of Pharmacy
Chapel Hill, North Carolina

Director
Department of Pharmacotherapy
South East Area Health Education
  Center (SEAHEC)
Wilmington, North Carolina

American Society of Health-System Pharmacists®
Bethesda, MD

Any correspondence regarding this publication should be sent to the publisher, American Society of Health-System Pharmacists, 7272 Wisconsin Avenue, Bethesda, MD 20814, attention: Special Publishing.

The information presented herein reflects the opinions of the contributors and advisors. It should not be interpreted as an official policy of ASHP or as an endorsement of any product. The information contained in this program, and the companion workbook, are to be used as guidance.

Because of ongoing research and improvements in technology, the information and its applications contained in this text are constantly evolving and are subject to the professional judgment and interpretation of the practitioner due to the uniqueness of each pharmacy's role in compounding sterile preparations and the handling of hazardous drugs. The editors, contributors, and ASHP have made reasonable efforts to ensure the accuracy and appropriateness of the information presented in this document. However, any user of this information is advised that the editors, contributors, advisors, and ASHP are not responsible for the continued currency of the information, for any errors or omissions, and/or for any consequences arising from the use of the information in the document in any and all practice settings. Any reader of this document is cautioned that ASHP makes no representation, guarantee, or warranty, express or implied, as to the accuracy and appropriateness of the information contained in this document and will bear no responsibility or liability for the results or consequences of its use.

Director, Special Publishing: Jack Bruggeman
Senior Editorial Project Manager: Dana Battaglia
Page Design: Carol Barrer

Library of Congress Cataloging-in-Publication Data

ASHP's clinical pearls / [edited by] Bruce Canaday.

p. ; cm.

Includes bibliographical references and index.

ISBN 978-1-58528-218-0

1. Clinical pharmacology--Case studies. I. Canaday, Bruce Robert. II. American Society of Health-System Pharmacists. III. ASHP Midyear Clinical Meeting (42nd : 2007 : Las Vegas, Nev.) IV. Title: Clinical pearls.

[DNLM: 1. Drug Therapy--Congresses. WB 330 A827 2008]

RM301.28.A84 2008

615'.1--dc22

2008038685

ISBN: 978-1-58528-218-0

# Contents

v     Note From the Publisher

vi    Preface

vii   Contributors

1      1— Potter's Pain: Harry, Hogwarts, and Headaches: Migraine Prophylaxis in an Adolescent and Young Adult Population
       *Daniel S. Longyhore*

9      2— My Life on the D-List: Clinical Importance of the Clindamycin-Inducible Resistance Test for *Staphylococcus aureus*
       *Joseph Kishel*

17     3—Getting the Knack of IV NAC: A Novel Dosing Strategy of N-acetylcysteine in a Patient Presenting with Severe Acetaminophen Toxicity
       *Erick J. Borkowski*

23     4— Pharmacy Proofs: $Cl_{cr} \neq GFR$
       *Jaime L. Borkowski*

31     5— Succinylcholine in the Critically Ill Patient: When Is It Not OK[+]?
       *Clyde Birringer*

35     6— Insulin Sliding Scales: To Use or Not to Use, That Is the Question
       *Jon Horton*

43     7— Glycemic Control in the ICU: How Low Should We Go?
       *Debra J. Skaar*

51      8—ASAP: Aspirin-Use Screen for Acute Myocardial Infarction Patients
        *Hoytin T. Lee Ghin*

55      9—Soy, You Want to be a Girlie Man? Effect of Soy Supplementation
        on Testosterone in Healthy Males
        *Susan Goodin*

63      10—Plan B Dosing for Plan B®: Alternative Dosing Strategies for
        Emergency Contraception with Levonorgestrel
        *Laura B. Hansen*

71      11—Warfarin and Cotrimoxazole: Averting Disaster
        *Todd R. Marcy*

79      12—Celiac Disease: Dangers of Gluten in Medications
        *Robert A. Magione*

87      13—Circumcision: Ouch!!
        *Rita K. Jew*

95      14—Friend or Foe? Ibuprofen for Patent Ductus Arteriosus
        *Allison Jun*

103     15—Hyporesponse to Erythropoietic Stimulating Agents:
        Uh-Oh, What Do We Do Now?
        *Sarah Tomasello*

123     Index

# Note from the Publisher

The Pearls sessions at the ASHP Midyear Clinical Meeting (MCM) are some of the best-attended sessions each year. With the publication of the "Pearls" series, ASHP is attempting to capture the best of these presentations with more in-depth coverage, which is not possible under the strict time constraints of the MCM pearls presentations. We hope you find this compilation worthwhile.

We encourage ASHP members to participate in the MCM Pearls presentations. To those who are participating in upcoming Pearl sessions, we hope you will consider turning those presentations into chapters for the Pearls book series. For additional information on becoming a Pearls series author, please contact me at jbruggeman@ashp.org

# Preface

A "Clinical Pearl" is intended to convey one idea, concept, fact, or other information that a clinician has found useful in day-to-day patient-care, but may not be widely known, understood, published, or taught.

Clinical Pearls are an ASHP tradition—beginning as a series of presentations at a "Midyear Clinical Meeting" in 1988 and continuing as the only educational program that has been offered at every winter meeting since that time. The success of these programs—they routinely attract some of the largest audiences at the meeting—likely relates to many factors: the expertise of the presenters, the value of the information, and the uniqueness of the format, both in brevity and in lightness of style.

Here for the first time, we have attempted to capture in book form the expertise, value, and brevity that characterized these traditional ASHP presentations. Selected presenters have been asked to expand on their original presentations at the ASHP Winter Meeting Clinical Pearls session to provide those who could not attend with the opportunity to access the information presented and to provide those who did attend more "depth" than was possible during the brief 5 minutes each speaker was afforded. So, whether you sat in on the session or not, there should be something useful for you in the pages that follow.

*Bruce Canaday*
*Clinical Professor and Vice-Chair*
*Division of Pharmacy Practice and Experiential Education*
*University of North Carolina, Eshelman School of Pharmacy*
*Chapel Hill, North Carolina*

*Director*
*Department of Pharmacotherapy*
*South East Area Health Education Center (SEAHEC)*
*Wilmington, North Carolina*

# Contributors

**Clyde Birringer, PharmD**
Clinical Specialist
Critical Care/Cardiology
Meriter Hospital Pharmacy Department
Madison, Wisconsin
cbirringer@meriter.com

**Erick J. Borkowski, PharmD**
Practice Coodinator/Clinical Pharmacist
Northwestern Memorial Hospital
Chicago, Illinois
 borko2@gmail.com

**Jaime L. Borkowski, PharmD, BCPS**
Pharmacy Clinical Coordinator
OSF St. Anthony Medical Center
Rockford, Illinois
Jaime.l.borkowski@ofshealthcare.org

**Hoytin T. Lee Ghin, PharmD, BCPS**
Clinical Assistant Professor Monmouth Medical Center
Ernest Mario School of Pharmacy
Rutgers University
Long Branch, New Jersey
erudition@hotmail.com

**Susan Goodin, PharmD, PharmD, FCCP, BCOP**
Director, Division of Pharmaceutical Sciences
The Cancer Institute of New Jersey
Professor of Medicine
UMDNJ, Robert Wood Johnson Medical School
New Brunswick, New Jersey
goodin@umdnj.edu

**Laura B. Hansen, PharmD, FCCP, BCPS**

Associate Professor

Departments of Clinical Pharmacology and Family Medicine

University of Colorado, Denver

School of Pharmacy

Aurora, Colorado

laura.hansen@uchsc.edu

**Jon Horton, PharmD, FASHP**

Clinical Pharmacy Manager

Director of Pharmacy Residency Programs

Department of Pharmacy

York Hospital

York, Pennsylvania

jhorton@wellspan.org

**Rita K. Jew, PharmD, FASHP**

Executive Director

Pharmacy Services

Children's Hospital of Orange County

Irvine, California

rjew@choc.org

**Allison Jun, PharmD**

Clinical Coordinator of Pharmacy Services

Neonatal Intensive Care Pharmacist

Children's Hospital of Orange County

Anaheim, California

aj_randle@yahoo.com

**Joseph Kishel, PharmD, BCPS**

Infectious Diseases Specialist, Milton S. Hershey Medical Center

Instructor of Pharmacology, Penn State College of Medicine

Hershey, PA

jkishel@psu.edu

**Daniel S. Longyhore, PharmD, BCPS**
Assistant Professor of Pharmacy Practice
Nesbitt College of Pharmacy and Nursing
Wilkes University
Wilkes Barre, Pennsylvania
longyhor@wilkes.edu

**Robert A. Mangione, RPh, EdD**
Dean and Clinical Professor
St. John's University College of Pharmacy and Allied Health Professions
Queens, New York
mangionr@stjohns.edu

**Todd R. Marcy, PharmD, BCPS, CDE**
Assistant Professor
University of Oklahoma
College of Pharmacy
Oklahoma City, Oklahoma
todd-marcy@ouhsc.edu

**Debra J. Skaar, PharmD**
Assistant Professor of Experimental and Clinical Pharmacology
Department of Experimental and Clinical Pharmacology
University of Minnesota College of Pharmacy
Minneapolis, Minnesota
skaar006@umn.edu

**Sarah Tomasello, PharmD, BCPS**
Clinical Associate Professor of Pharmacy
Ernest Mario School of Pharmacy
Rutgers, The State University of New Jersey
Piscataway, New Jersey
Clinical Specialist – Nephrology
Robert Wood Johnson University Hospital
New Brunswick, New Jersey
stomasel@rci.rutgers.edu

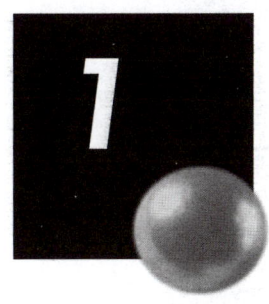

# Potter's Pain: Harry, Hogwarts, and Headaches: Migraine Prophylaxis in an Adolescent and Young Adult Population

*Daniel S. Longyhore*

## Clinical Scenario

H. Potter is a 17-year-old male complaining of worsening headaches over the last 3 years. He states that his headaches were infrequent, short, and only slightly painful prior to his 15th birthday. However, since then, he has noticed that the frequency and severity of the headaches has increased greatly. Currently, the pain is the worst it has ever been and is enough to "knock him off his feet." The headaches are beginning to affect his schoolwork, quality of life, and even his activities of daily living. He cannot identify a physical, auditory, or olfactory trigger for the headaches, but they usually present when he becomes psychologically connected with He-Who-Must-Not-Be-Named (Lord Voldemort).[1]

## Introduction

Headaches affect a vast number of individuals annually, accounting for approximately 10 million family medicine and neurology visits each year.[2] Of these, migraine headaches are the second most prevalent type of headache, but may be considered the most debilitating. It is estimated that the 1-year incidence of migraine headaches may be as high as 15% in the American and European populations.[3] The World Health Organization ranks migraine headaches as the nineteenth most disabling disease worldwide.[4]

A number of renowned individuals have been noted to suffer from migraine headaches, including Vincent Van Gogh. At the time of his ailment, headache disorders were not well understood, and Van Gogh was readily diagnosed as having a psychiatric illness, for which he was hospitalized and treated. During one hospitalization in Paris, France, Van Gogh painted the famous *Starry Night*. The picture is speculated to be the view from his hospital window.

More recently in popular culture, J.K. Rowling's character Harry Potter was passively evaluated for his recurring head pain. In an article by Dr. Sheftell and colleagues,[5] Mr. Potter's headaches and accompanying symptoms throughout the first six books of the seven book series were reviewed to potentially diagnose his headache disorder. The researchers were able to identify all but one of the necessary International Classification of Headache Disorders – Second Edition

## Table 1.1. International Headache Society: The International Classification of Headache Disorders Migraine Headache Diagnostic Criteria

I.      At least 5 attacks fulfilling criteria II through IV.

II.     Headache attack lasting 4-72 hours (untreated or unsuccessfully treated)

III.    Headache has at least 2 of the following characteristics:

    a. Unilateral location

    b. Pulsating quality

    c. Moderate or severe pain intensity

    d. Aggravation by or causing avoidance of routine physical activity (e.g., walking or climbing stairs)

IV.     During headache at least one of the following:

    a. Nausea and/or vomiting

    b. Photophobia and/or phonophobia

V.      Not attributed to any other disorder

## Table 1.2. Suggested Patients to Receive Migraine Headache Prophylaxis

- Two or more attacks per month
- Recurring migraines that, in the patient's opinion, significantly interfere with their daily routines, despite acute treatment
- Frequent headaches
- Contradiction to, failure of, or overuse of acute therapies
- Adverse events with acute therapies
- Excess cost for both acute and preventative therapies
- Patient preference
- The presence of uncommon migraine conditions, including hemiplegic migraine, basilar migraine, migraine with prolonged aura, or migrainous infarction (to prevent neurologic damage – as based on expert consensus)

(ICHD-II) criteria for migraine headaches, leading to the diagnosis of 1.6 *Probable Migraine* (Table 1.1).[6] Do his headaches warrant therapy beyond abortive migraine therapy, though?

The United States Headache Consortium established parameters for prophylaxis based on migraine headache frequency and severity (Table 1.2).[7] These criteria should be viewed as suggestions for initiating agents for prophylaxis and are flexible in their interpretation.

Emphasis should be placed on the criteria of "patient preference," given that even infrequent migraine headaches of debilitating proportions may be enough to warrant preventing future attacks. There are multiple agents recommended by the US Headache Consortium first line for prophylaxis of migraine headaches, including amitriptyline, propranolol, and divalproex. Since this publication in 2000, topiramate has also proven efficacy in decreasing the frequency and severity of migraine headaches. At target doses, these agents are effective in a majority of patients with migraine headaches. Unfortunately, these medications have various limitations to use, as well.

The common adverse event profile associated with most of the first line agents may deter patients from wanting to use them appropriately and push them to target doses. These adverse events may be especially concerning in young children and adolescents, like the students of Hogwart's School of Witchcraft and Wizardry.[1] In a setting where certain medications may alter attentiveness, concentration, and body habitus, children and adolescents may be less likely to use medications and attempt to just deal with the migraine headache pain.[8]

In the case presented at the beginning of the chapter, H. Potter complained of headaches of worsening frequency and intensity. And, according to Dr. Sheftell and colleagues, the symptomatic presentation across the first six published works was enough to diagnose Harry with *probable migraine*. The next step would then be to evaluate Harry's need for migraine headache prophylaxis based on his symptoms and frequency of symptoms. While the exact quantity of migraine headaches is not reported, it is stated that Harry's headaches significantly impact his life and functionality. According to the US Headache Consortium, if Harry's preference were to not experience the headaches and their debilitating nature, it would be sufficient to warrant migraine headache prophylaxis.

## Therapy

As with most disease states, the use of non-pharmacologic measures should be encouraged with medications to prevent migraine headaches. Migraineurs should avoid potential triggers such as nitrate- and tyramine-containing foods and beverages, avoid potent olfactory stimuli, and/or decrease stress. In the case of Harry Potter, his migraine trigger was (many times) unavoidable because of the mystical connection he shared with Lord Voldemort. He was unable to avoid the trigger just as a person whose trigger is strong perfume may find it difficult to avoid persons who wear too much perfume. In situations like this, medication is ideal to help prevent migraine headaches because of the unpredictability of migraine headache onset. Table 1.3 lists the commonly used migraine headache prophylaxis agents by their efficacy and adverse event profile.

Amitriptylline (and nortriptylline by association) is regarded as an effective agent for migraine headache prophylaxis at doses of 50 to 150 mg (25 to 75 mg for nortriptyline). Taken at bedtime, this agent has the potential to reduce migraine headache frequency. However, the adverse event profile is less than ideal, and at higher doses, may cause excessive or prolonged sedation and metabolic changes and/or weight gain.[9] This is a two-fold fault with the agent for adolescents like Harry Potter, especially because the excessive and sometimes prolonged sedation may effect the student's classroom performance. As well, the more image-conscious adolescents become, the addition of 3 to 5 pounds may be enough of a deterrent for using a tricyclic antidepressant to prevent migraine headaches. In the world of Harry Potter, the use of tricyclic antidepres-

## Table 1.3. Preventative Therapy Options for Migraine Headaches

| Quality of Evidence A* | Quality of Evidence B† | Quality of Evidence C†† |
|---|---|---|
| *Antiepileptics* | | |
| Divalproate | Carbamazepine | |
| Topiramate* | Gabapentin | |
| *Antidepressants* | | |
| Amitriptyline | Fluoxetine | Nortriptyline |
| | | Imipramine |
| *Beta-blockers* | | |
| Propranolol | Atenolol | |
| Timolol | Nadolol | |
| | Metoprolol | |
| *Calcium Channel Blockers* | | |
| | Nimodipine | Diltiazem |
| | Verapamil | |
| *Other Agents* | | |
| | Feverfew | |
| | Magnesium | |
| | Vitamin B2 (riboflavin) | |

*Quality of Evidence A: Multiple well-designed randomized clinical trials, directly relevant to the recommendation, yielded a consistent pattern of findings.

†Quality of Evidence B: Some evidence from randomized clinical trials supported the recommendation, but the scientific support was not optimal. For instance, either few randomized trials existed, the trials that did exist were somewhat inconsistent, or the trials were not directly relevant to the recommendation.[11–14]

††Quality of Evidence C: The US Headache Consortium achieved consensus on the recommendation in the absence of relevant randomized controlled trials.

sants may be more harmful than beneficial, regardless of the migraine headache benefit. Harry may find himself having difficulty concentrating during classes, napping in the early evening instead of doing his classwork, or having trouble staying awake in class. The medication may be dosed in the evening, with hopes that he will sleep through most of the adverse events, but the side effects may last into the daytime. Adolescents, whether muggle or wizard, have the tendency to be quite image conscious and even the threat of weight gain when starting a new medication may deter a patient from remaining adherent to the drug.

The use of beta-blockers, specifically propranolol, is also considered a first line agent to prevent migraine headaches. Although this agent may be an appropriate choice for an adult patient with concurrent cardiovascular disease, its adverse event profile may be troublesome to children and adolescents, especially those who are highly active or have respiratory disease, such as asthma. The use of the beta receptor antagonist may offer the ability to decrease Harry's migraine headache frequency and severity, but it may also affect his athletic performance and cause premature fatigue.[10] Harry Potter is an avid Quidditch player, who requires a certain level of physical exertion to play well. Harry is the Seeker and is constantly required to be attentive to his surroundings to duck and dodge quickly and effectively. In the presence of a beta-blocker, Harry may experience early fatigue or delayed recovery times because his heart is unable to keep up with the oxygen demands of his body. As well, [WARNING: book spoiler] Harry may not have been victorious in his battles with Lord Voldemort had he been physically hampered by the presence of propranolol.

Antiepileptic agents, such as divalproex and topiramate, have also proven efficacious for the prevention of migraine headaches. However, like the previously mentioned agents, they also carry with them adverse event profiles that could be less ideal for adolescent patients. While topiramate use may be associated with a slight weight loss, it is also capable of causing prolonged daytime sedation at the doses necessary to prevent migraine headaches (100-200 mg daily).[11] Divalproex's downfalls are much the same as the tricyclic antidepressants in that it may cause weight gain and/or hair loss in a demographic that is very image conscious.[9] Many of these adverse events have been discussed previously and how they may affect Harry Potter's academic performance, if utilized.

The adverse events of the previously mentioned agents and the potential to decrease adolescent patient adherence puts providers in a peculiar predicament. How should a young patient like Mr. Potter with migraine headaches that affect both academic and social situation, as well as cause a great deal of pain, be managed efficiently? For that answer, more attention should be focused toward the second line options for preventing migraine headaches, including verapamil, magnesium, and vitamin B2 (riboflavin).[15] These agents have evidence to support a trial in a patient population that needs migraine headache prevention without extra adverse events. While some of the agents that were previously accepted as alternatives to first line therapies are falling out of favor due to questionable evidence, others continue to build their case and show their benefit as options for migraine headache prevention.

Historically, verapamil was considered the agent of choice for athletes with migraine headaches. Verapamil was thought to have the benefit of preventing or decreasing migraine headache severity without affecting athletic endurance like propranolol and other beta receptor antagonists. However, while some clinical trials suggest that there is a benefit for migraine prevention, other trials have shown high dropout rates because of adverse.[2,3] When visualizing the potential risks and benefits that Harry Potter would receive from this agent, it appears that the risk of adverse events is greater than the perceived benefit. As previously stated, the reported efficacy of verapamil has been brought into question and many more practitioners are avoiding the medication because it may not work. So, while verapamil may still have a role in preventing migraine headaches, it is with less convincing evidence and a continued risk of adverse events. And while an option, it is not a preferred second line option.

Magnesium supplementation is commonly overlooked as a viable over-the-counter alternative for migraine headache prophylaxis. At doses of 500 mg daily, magnesium may decrease the frequency and severity of migraine headaches. Most patients should be able to use magnesium without increased risk of adverse events, except for those with compromised renal function. In fact, some patient populations, specifically pregnant women, may consider magnesium as a first line agent given its low risk for teratogenicity and frequent use in premature contractions. Controlling migraine headaches can be difficult in the pregnant population because increased teratogenic risk with antidepressant and anticonvulsant use. As well, many of the abortive agents pose a risk to the maturing fetus. A supplement such as magnesium that may provide relief from migraine headaches without increasing the changes of fetal damage or terminating the pregnancy would be ideal. In the case of Harry, magnesium use may decrease his migraine headache severity and frequency, without the potential of adverse event. As a young white male, the chances of having compromised renal function are low. The only adverse event that is common with oral magnesium therapy is diarrhea. Clinical trials have reported as many as 45.7% of patients (versus 23.5% of placebo patients) reporting diarrhea during treatment.[14]

Like magnesium, riboflavin offers an over-the-counter alternative to migraine headache prophylaxis with a less serious adverse event profile. The effective dose of riboflavin is 400 mg daily. Research reports that at this dose, migraine headache frequency and severity are reduced by at least 50% in 59% or more of patients.[5] As stated, the adverse event profile of riboflavin is relatively benign, with the worst adverse event being urine discoloration (yellow-orange). At these doses, European research has reported diarrhea and polyuria as adverse events, but they were not more common than adverse events reported by those taking placebo.

## Conclusion

In review, Harry Potter's (probable) migraine headaches are frequent and severe enough to warrant daily prophylactic therapy. The therapy chosen should be not only effective, but cause less adverse drug reactions to avoid nonadherence with therapy. The current first line agents such as antidepressants, antiepileptics, and antihypertensives have good evidence to support their use, but their adverse events may be a burden to an aspiring wizard. In this case, a second line agent with less adverse events would be ideal. Verapamil has less performance effects, but its efficacy for preventing migraine headaches is being called into question. Magnesium offers much of the same efficacy and is only limited by causing diarrhea in approximately 50% of patients treated with it. Vitamin B2 (riboflavin) appears to be the best choice given its efficacy data and adverse event profile similar to placebo. The use of riboflavin 400 mg daily by Harry Potter should noticeably decrease his migraine headaches without affecting his busy activities of daily living at Hogwart's School of Witchcraft and Wizardry.

## References

1. Rowling JK. *Harry Potter* series. New York, NY; Scholastic Publishing: 1998 through 2007.
2. Ramadan NM, Silberstein SD, Freitag FG, et al. Evidence-based guidelines for migraine headache in the primary care setting: pharmacological management for prevention of migraine. 2000. Available online at http://www.aan.com/professionals/practice/guidelines. cfm. Accessed March 20, 2008.

3. Headache Disorders and Public Health; Education and Management Implications. WHO/MSD/MBD/OO.9 2000. Available online at http:// www.migraines.org/new/pdfs/who.pdf. Accessed March 20, 2008.

4. The International Classification of Headache Disorders. *Cephalagia* 2004;23:Suppl 1.

5. Sheftell F, Steiner TJ, Thomas H. Harry Potter and the Curse of Headache. *Headache* 2007;47:911-916.

6. Headache Classification Subcommittee on the International Headache Society. The International Classification of Headache Disorders, 2nd edition. *Cephalalgia* 2004;24:(Suppl 1):1-160.

7. Ramadan NM, Silberstein SD, Freitag FG, et al. Evidence Based Guidelines for Migraine Headache in the Primary Care Setting: Pharmacological Management for Prevention of Migraine. Available online at http://www.neurology.org. Accessed March 21, 2008.

8. Matsui D. Current Issues in Pediatric Medication Adherence. *Pediatric Drugs* 2007;9:283-288.

9. Maggioni F, Ruffatti S, Dianese F, et al. Weight variations in the prophylaxis of primary headaches: a 6-month follow-up. *J Headache Pain* 2005;6:322-324.

10. Niedfeldt MW. Managing hypertension in athletes and physically active patients. *Am Fam Phys* 2002;66:445-452.

11. Brandes JL, Saper JR, Diamond M, et al. Topiramate for migraine prevention. *JAMA* 2007;291:965-973.

12. Modi S, Lowder DM. Medications for Migraine Prophylaxis. *Am Fam Phys* 2006;73:72-78.

13. Ramadan NM, Silberstein SD, Freitag FG, et al. Evidence-based guidelines for migraine headache in the primary care setting: pharmacological management for prevention of migraine. Available online at http://www.aan.com/professionals/practice/guideline. Accessed March 21, 2008.

14. Pfafferath V, Wessely P, Meyer C, et al. Magnesium in the prophylaxis of migraine—A double-blind, placebo-controlled study. *Cephalalgia* 1996;16:436-440.

15. Schoenen J, Jacquy J, Lenaerts M. Effectiveness of high-dose riboflavin in migraine prophylaxis: A randomized controlled trial. *Neurology* 1998;50:466-470.

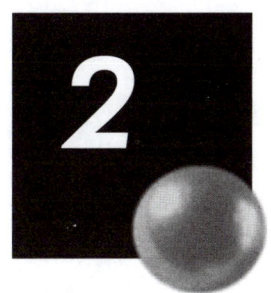

# 2

# My Life on the D-List: Clinical Importance of the Clindamycin-Inducible Resistance Test for *Staphylococcus aureus*

*Joseph Kishel*

## Background

### Development of Community-Associated Methicillin-Resistant Staphylococcus aureus

Methicillin-resistant *Staphylococcus aureus* (MRSA) is an important pathogen and significant healthcare issue, which has gained significant notoriety even in the lay press.[1] The first isolates of MRSA were identified in the United Kingdom in 1961, with subsequent isolates identified in the United States and then worldwide after 1968.[2,3] Not surprising to contemporary clinicians, methicillin resistance manifested shortly after the introduction of methicillin to the anti-bacterial armamentarium. The tale of MRSA continues to evolve; prevalence of MRSA in US hospitals has been steadily increasing since the 1980s and has only started to plateau with aggressive infection control procedures, such as contact isolation for infected patients and hand washing initiatives for healthcare workers. As MRSA rates in US hospitals approach 60% or greater, a new threat has emerged: community-associated MRSA (CA-MRSA).

Initial reports of CA-MRSA were in patients not normally associated with drug resistant bacterial infections: pre-teen and teenage adolescents and professional athletes. Other case reports included patients living in community settings (e.g., military personnel, prisoners), men who have sex with men, and tattoo recipients.[4–6] Despite the abundance of case data regarding the epidemiology of CA-MRSA, risk factors for infection with these bacteria are not well defined. Because of the prevalence and community awareness of CA-MRSA, most emergency room or family practice physicians are now familiar with the presentation of CA-MRSA skin and skin structure infections. This awareness may be due to the distinctive nature of the presenting symptoms, chronicity of the disease, potential for morbidity and mortality upon dissemination, and increasing incidence of MRSA with a community source. CA-MRSA incidence varies geographically (ranging from 5 to 95%); however, most experts agree that a 50% incidence of CA-MRSA in the US emergency rooms is a fair estimate.[7] A common chief complaint is what look like spider bites or

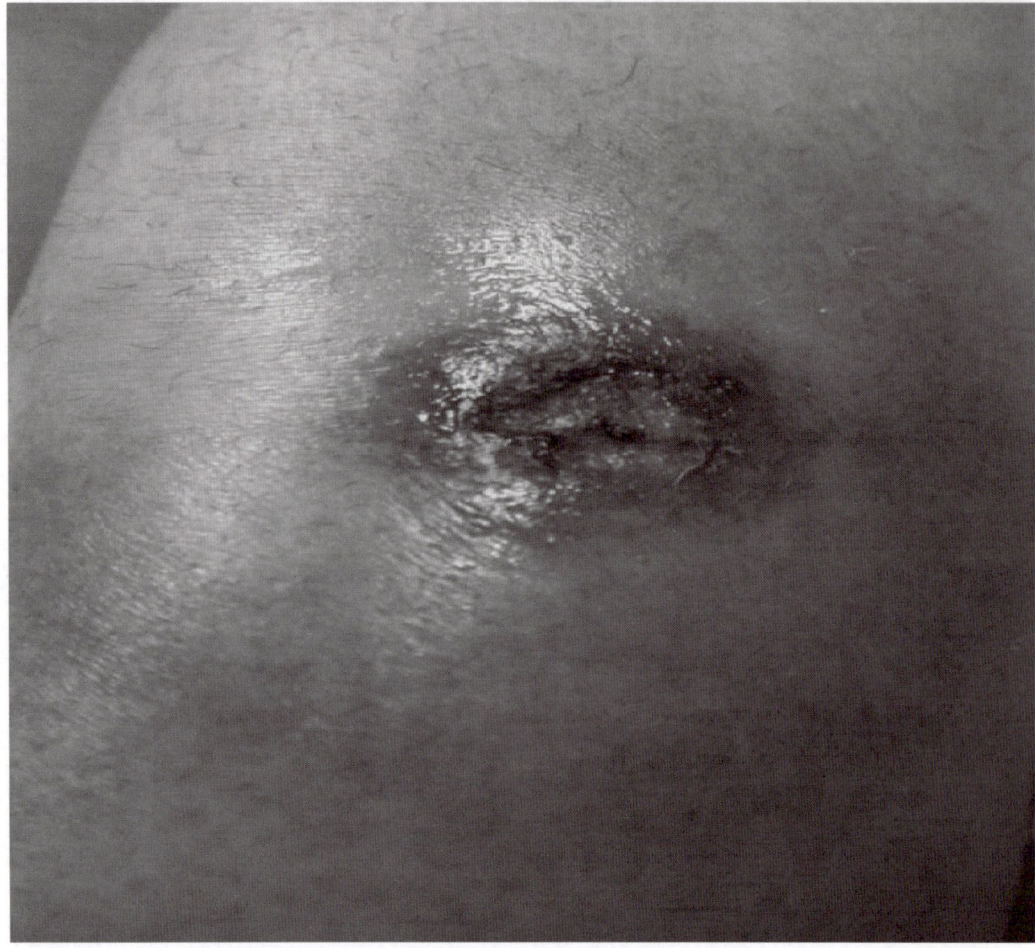

**Figure 2.1.** Brown recluse spider bite. Reprinted with permission from Casey, Mold: The clinical characteristics of brown recluse spider bites treated by family physicians. *J Fam Pract* 1999;48:7.

multiple lesions that can be anywhere on the surface of the skin, some purulent, some with a necrotic center (Fig. 2.1). Despite the limited geographic distribution of biting spiders such as the brown recluse (Loxescles spp), the complaint of "spider bite" persists. The trained physician knows to consider CA-MRSA in the differential of a patient presenting with multiple skin abscesses. The remaining patients presenting with CA-MRSA often have much more serious disease, manifesting as CA-MRSA pneumonia. Previously, Staphylococcal pneumonia was rather uncommon; presenting only as a secondary infection after viral influenza. Today, MRSA is a recognizable cause of hospital-acquired pneumonia, ventilator-associated pneumonia, and CA-MRSA pneumonia. In many cases, this pneumonia is necrotizing and causes significant morbidity and mortality in patients who were otherwise healthy prior to disease presentation.

## Mechanisms of Resistance

*Staphylococcus aureus* develops resistance to methicillin, and by extension all beta lactam type antibiotics (with the exception of the investigational antibiotic ceftibiprole), via the *mecA* gene which codes for the altered penicillin receptor binding protein 2a (PBP2a). Presence of the *mecA* gene yields MRSA.[8] Resistance to macrolides can occur through multiple mechanisms. The gene *msrA* codes for an efflux pump causing erythromycin resistance. The ribosomal target for macrolides, lincosamides, and streptogramins can be altered by the gene *erm*, this alteration can be constitutive or inducible.[9] Constitutive resistance is detectable with standard antimicrobial susceptibility testing; inducible resistance will only manifest in the presence of an inducer, and requires additional testing.

## Pharmacotherapy for CA-MRSA

Antimicrobial treatment of MRSA is further complicated by the lack of antibiotics available to treat infections due to this organism. When considering antibiosis for the patient, it is important to consider the nature of the infection as well as the source of the bacteria. It is not in the scope of this chapter to discuss principles and practices of infectious diseases as it pertains to site of infection. A more focused consideration for discussion here is to recognize the nature of the MRSA infection and rationally determine an appropriate antibiotic regimen. Although they share resistance to methicillin, CA-MRSA and Hospital Associated-MRSA (HA-MRSA) are not the same entity. These bacteria differ in pathogenicity, predilection for disease site, genotypic make-up, and phenotypic expression of this genotype as it pertains to antimicrobial susceptibility.[10,11] In the treatment of an HA-MRSA most clinicians would consider vancomycin as a first line antibiotic in the hospitalized patient. Other antimicrobials such as daptomycin, dalfopristin/quinupristin, doxycycline, linezolid, sulfamethoxazole/trimethoprim, and tigecycline usually have activity against HA-MRSA and may be preferred over vancomycin in certain disease states and certain situations. CA-MRSA is often susceptible to the same antibiotics as HA-MRSA, but is often also susceptible to ciprofloxacin, erythromycin, and clindamycin. The clinical utility of ciprofloxacin and erythromycin in the treatment of MRSA infections is minimal to non-existent; however the susceptibility data are often useful in differentiating CA-MRSA from HA-MRSA in the absence of better data. The utility of incision and debridement for an abscess must not be discounted (the surgeon's mantra of "If there is an abscess, drain it!" holds true here). Given that a physician would generally prefer not to treat an outpatient with a cellulitis or abscess due to MRSA with an intravenous antibiotic, the utility of an oral antibiotic becomes paramount. As previously discussed, as much as 50% of outpatient Staphylococcal skin infections may be due to CA-MRSA. As with other infections, there can be a high penalty for initially choosing inappropriate antibiotics.[12] These outpatients are often treated with oral sulfamethoxazole/trimethoprim, optimally at a weight based – not UTI – dose, and sent home. However, due to renal dysfunction or allergy, sulfa drugs are sometimes not an option. Clindamycin is a useful alternative in the oral management of CA-MRSA skin infections, given good oral bioavailability, low cost, and reasonable side effect profile. However, the nature of CA-MRSA resistance requires caution in empiric use of clindamycin without antibiotic susceptibility data.

# Clinical Significance of Inducible Clindamycin Resistance

## The Scope of Clindamycin Resistance

Three situations bear discussion here. The first is in the setting of a Staphylococcal species isolate that is erythromycin susceptible and clindamycin susceptible. In this situation, clindamycin would be a clinically rational choice, given no other negative patient considerations. The second situation is in the setting of erythromycin resistance and clindamycin resistance. This situation is described as constitutive ribosomal alteration (macrolide lincosamide streptogramin B constitutive - $MLS_bc$) by the *erm* gene, and thus clindamycin would not be clinically useful in this setting. This situation would be accurately detected by standard antimicrobial susceptibility testing. The third situation is a Staphylococcal species isolate that is erythromycin resistant, but is determined to be clindamycin susceptible by standard antimicrobial susceptibility testing. Further investigation is necessary in this situation due to the mechanism of erythromycin resistance. Again, this resistance is coded by the *erm* gene, however, resistance is expressed in an inducible nature ($MLS_bi$) – meaning exposure to the antibiotic of interest yields resistance. The clinical relevance of this situation is a patient who appears to be susceptible to clindamycin, is prescribed this drug for the infection of interest, and then fails therapy. The patient fails therapy because the use of clindamycin in the setting of an inducible *erm* gene quickly confers resistance to clindamycin resulting in clinical failure. This situation has been described in numerous case reports.[13–15] It is important to note that we use erythromycin resistance as a surrogate marker for this phenomenon; the patient does not require receipt of erythromycin then clindamycin in succession for clinical or microbiological failure to occur.

## Testing for Clindamycin-Inducible Resistance

Standard antimicrobial susceptibility testing fails to detect $MLS_bi$ strains of Staphylococci. The Clindamycin Disk Induction Test for *Staphylococcus* spp (aka the "D test" so named for the "D" shape noted on a positive test) was developed to clinically test for this phenomenon. To perform this test, isolates are plated on a Mueller-Hinton agar plate at a MacFarland concentration of 0.5 to evenly cover the agar surface. Clindamycin and erythromycin disks, containing 2 mcg and 15 mcg of each antibiotic, respectively, are placed in the center of the plate separated by a distance of 1.5 cm between the edges. Plates are incubated at 37°C for 24 hours. Inducible resistance to clindamycin was defined as blunting of the clear circular area of no growth around the clindamycin disk on the side adjacent to the erythromycin disk and was designated D-test positive. Absence of a blunted zone of inhibition was designated D-test negative, which shows that the strain is truly susceptible to clindamycin Figure 2.2.[16]

## Recommendations for Use of the Clindamycin Disk Induction Test

The Clindamycin Disk Induction Test for Staphylococcus spp should be performed to confer accurate data about the utility of clindamycin in the setting of erythromycin resistance. At our facility, this test is automatically performed on Staphylococcus spp isolates from skin sources, and on beta hemolytic Group B Streptococcus vaginal screening isolates, the latter being per-

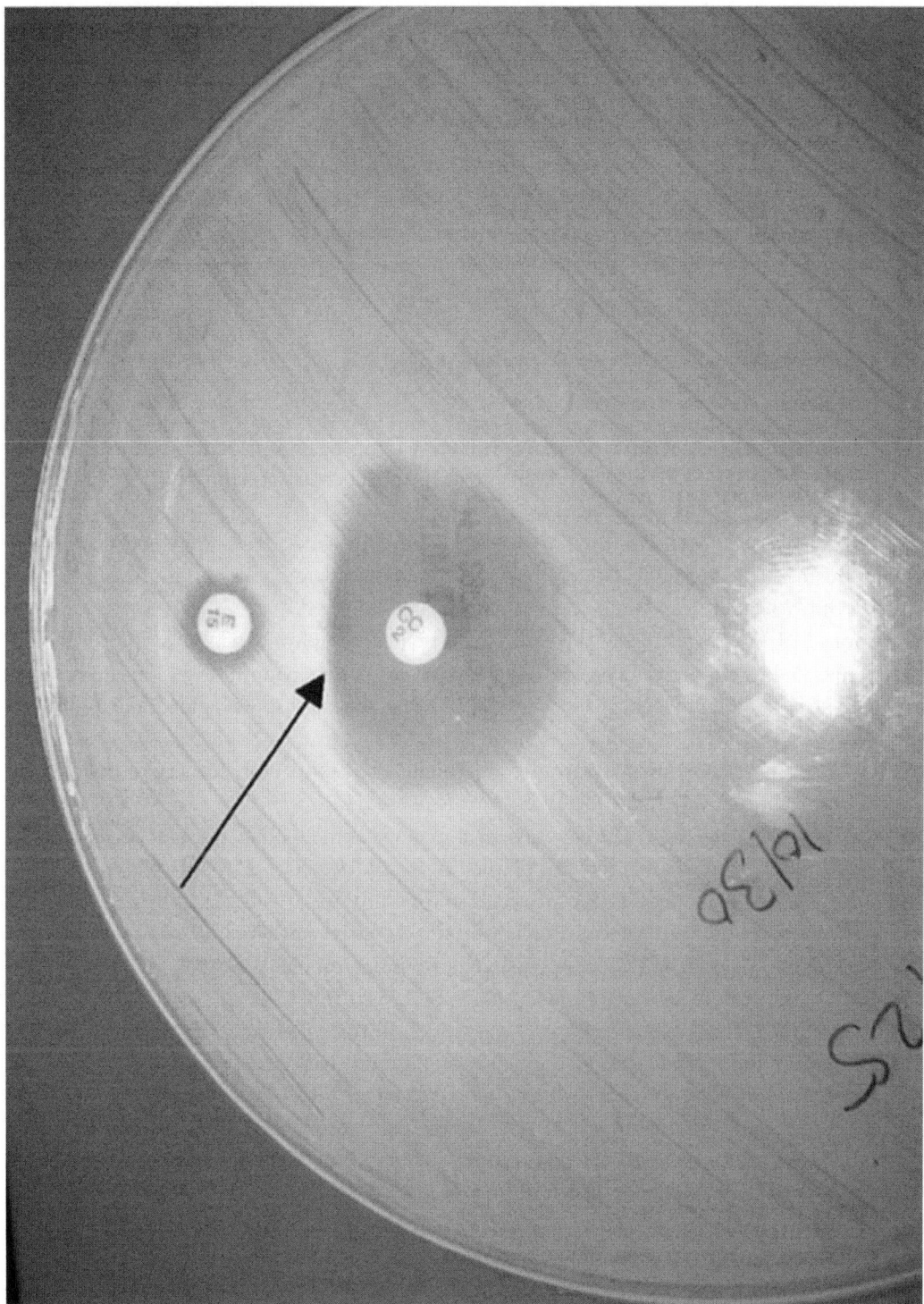

**Figure 2.2.** Positive "D test." Note the "D" shaped blunting of the Clindamycin Zone of inhibition. Reprinted with permission from Siberry GK, Tekle T, Carroll K, et al. Failure of clindamycin treatment of methicillin-resistant *Staphylococcus aureus* expressing inducible clindamycin resistance in vitro. *Clin Infect Dis* 2003;37:1257-60.

formed pre-delivery where the utility of clindamycin is paramount in the GBS (+) pregnant woman who is penicillin allergic.

## Summary

The Clindamycin Disk Induction Test for Staphylococcus spp (or "D test") is a subtlety of infectious diseases pharmacotherapy. The importance of obtaining this test and properly interpreting the results of this test can have important implications in the patient with a Staphylococcal or Streptococcal infection in whom clindamycin is being considered.

## References

1. "Superbug" MRSA Worries Doctors, Athletes: Drug-Resistant Germ Found in Locker Rooms; Can Kill Within Days. Available at: http://abcnews.go.com/Health/Primetime/Story?id=410908&page=1. Accessed April 3, 2008.

2. Barrett FF, McGehee RF, Jr., Finland M. Methicillin-resistant Staphylococcus aureus at Boston City Hospital. Bacteriologic and epidemiologic observations. *N Engl J Med* 1968;279:441-8.

3. Jevons MP, Coe AW, Parker MT. Methicillin resistance in staphylococci. *Lancet* 1963;1:904-7.

4. Benjamin HJ, Nikore V, Takagishi J. Practical management: community-associated methicillin-resistant Staphylococcus aureus (CA-MRSA): the latest sports epidemic. *Clin J Sport Med* 2007;17:393-7.

5. Lu D, Holtom P. Community-acquired methicillin-resistant Staphylococcus aureus, a new player in sports medicine. *Curr Sports Med Rep* 2005;4:265-70.

6. Kazakova SV, Hageman JC, Matava M, et al. A clone of methicillin-resistant *Staphylococcus aureus* among professional football players. *N Engl J Med* 2005;352:468--75.

7. Community-Associated MRSA Information for Clinicans. Available at: http://www.cdc.gov/ncidod/dhqp/ar_mrsa_ca_clinicians.html. Accessed April 3, 2008.

8. Hartman BJ, Tomasz A. Low-affinity penicillin-binding protein associated with beta-lactam resistance in Staphylococcus aureus. *J Bacteriol* 1984;158:513-6.

9. Weisblum B. Inducible resistance to macrolides, lincosamides and streptogramin type B antibiotics: the resistance phenotype, its biological diversity, and structural elements that regulate expression--a review. *J Antimicrob Chemother* 1985;16Suppl A:63-90.

10. Martinez-Aguilar G, Hammerman WA, Mason EO Jr, Kaplan SL. Clindamycin treatment of invasive infections caused by community acquired, methicillin-resistant and methicillin-susceptible Staphylococcus aureus in children. *Pediatr Infect Dis J* 2003;22:593–598.

11. Naimi TS, LeDell KH, Boxrud DJ, et al. Epidemiology and clonality of community-acquired methicillin-resistant Staphylococcus aureus in Minnesota, 1996–1998. *Clin Infect Dis* 2001;33:990 –996.

12. Kollef MH, Ward S, Sherman G, et al. Inadequate treatment of nosocomial infections is associated with certain empiric antibiotic choices. *Crit Care Med* 2000;28:3456-3464.

13. Huang H, Flynn NM, King JH, et al. Comparisons of community-associated methicillin-resistant Staphylococcus aureus (MRSA) and hospital-associated MSRA infections in Sacramento, California. *J Clin Microbiol* 2006;44:2423-2427.

14. Siberry GK, Tekle T, Carroll K, Dick J. Failure of clindamycin treatment of methicillin-resistant Staphylococcus aureus expressing inducible clindamycin resistance in vitro. *Clin Infect Dis* 2003;37:1257-1260.

15. Levin TP, Suh B, Axelrod P, et al. Potential clindamycin resistance in clindamycin-susceptible, erythromycin-resistant Staphylococcus aureus: report of a clinical failure. *Antimicrob Agents Chemother* 2005;49:1222-1224.

16. NCCLS. 2004. Performance standards for antimicrobial susceptibility testing: 14th informational supplement. NCCLS document M100-S14. NCCLS, Wayne, PA.

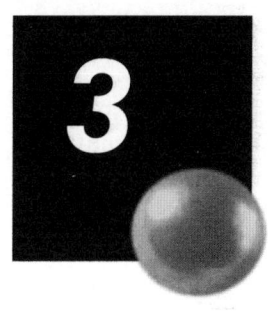

# 3

# Getting the Knack of IV NAC: A Novel Dosing Strategy of N-acetylcysteine in a Patient Presenting with Severe Acetaminophen Toxicity

*Erick J. Borkowski*

## Background

The use of acetylcysteine to treat hepatotoxicity as a result of acetaminophen overdose was first described in 1974 by Matthew and Prescott.[1] Today, almost 35 years later, controversy still exists in how to treat the acetaminophen overdose patient due in large part to a lack of studies comparing various regimens. Various strategies including the use of oral or intravenous (IV) N-acetylcysteine (NAC) at different doses and durations of treatment are described in the literature. The case report below describes a strategy that is not clearly defined in the literature but is recommended by the Illinois Poison Control Center.

## Institution

The following case occurred at an 897 bed, level I trauma, academic hospital located in downtown Chicago, Illinois. The hospital sees over 70,000 emergency department visits annually as well as over 40,000 inpatient admissions.

## Case

In October 2006, a 24-year-old female was brought to the emergency department after being found in the hallway outside of her home by the Chicago Fire Department. In the emergency department, it was ascertained that the patient had a history of prior suicide attempts. She was disoriented and incoherent and told the staff she believed she was having a miscarriage. She admitted to acetaminophen ingestion in combination with alcohol although she was unable to describe how much acetaminophen or alcohol was consumed. In addition, she was unable to tell the staff how long it had been since she consumed the acetaminophen and alcohol. Her medication history was otherwise unremarkable. She was tachycardic, hypotensive (70/40 mm

Hg), and hypothermic (91°F). She was resuscitated with 6 L of IV fluid and started on broad spectrum antibiotics, norepinephrine, and vasopressin. She was intubated for impending respiratory failure, and IV NAC was initiated at a dose of 150 mg/kg over 15 minutes, followed by 50 mg/kg over 4 hours, and finally 100 mg/kg over 16 hours. This final dose of NAC was repeated every 16 hours in the intensive care unit (ICU) for a total IV NAC length of therapy of 101 hours. In the ICU, her acetaminophen level was 50.0 μg/mL (therapeutic range = 10-25 μg/mL), alcohol level was 63 mg/dL, ammonia was 217μmol/L (normal range = 0-59 μmol/L), hemoglobin was 8.4 g/dL (normal range = 11.6-15.4 g/dL), platelets were 107,000/μL (normal range = 140,00-390,000/ μL), INR was 9.9 (normal range = 0.9- 1.2), and alanine aminotransferase/aspartate aminotransferase (ALT/AST) were 4077 units/L (normal range = 0-48) and 29049 units/L (normal range = 0-40), respectively.

## Mechanism of Action of Acetaminophen Toxicity

When acetaminophen is consumed, approximately 4% of the drug is metabolized to the potentially toxic N-acetyl-p-benzoquinoneimine (NAPQI) via the cytochrome P-450 system.[1] Under normal physiologic conditions, this metabolite will bind with glutathione to form nontoxic cysteine and mercapturic acid. In the patient presenting with acetaminophen overdose, a much greater quantity of acetaminophen must be metabolized through this pathway, depleting glutathione stores and increasing the concentration of NAPQI. It is this unconjugated NAPQI that is responsible for the hepatic damage that occurs.

## Mechanism of Action of N-acetylcysteine

Acetylcysteine is the nonproprietary name for the N-acetyl derivative of the naturally occurring amino acid, L-cysteine (N-acetyl-L-cysteine, NAC).[2] NAC appears to act as an antidote in acetaminophen overdose in two ways. First, NAC prevents NAPQI from binding to hepatocytes, preventing liver toxicity.[1] Second, L-cysteine is essential for glutathione production, and NAC acts by providing L-cysteine for the stimulation of glutathione synthesis.[3] By both binding to NAPQI itself and assisting in the production and repletion of glutathione stores, NAC can be effective in treating the acetaminophen overdose patient.

## Dosing of N-acetylcysteine

There are a number of regimens that differ in route of administration, dose, and duration of therapy as described in the literature for NAC.4-6 Additionally, a nomogram has been developed to predict the likelihood of hepatotoxicity and to help practitioners decide whether NAC is warranted.7 Although opinions vary regarding when to use oral or IV and what dosing regimen to use, there is consensus that the sooner NAC is started, the better the chance of avoiding severe hepatotoxicity. The best outcomes are seen when NAC is started no later than 10 and preferably within 8 hours post acetaminophen ingestion, regardless of the route of administration, dose, or duration of therapy.3 Although early administration of NAC is preferable, treatment is still recommended in patients who present greater than 10 hours post ingestion.

The current Food and Drug Administration (FDA)- approved dosing of IV NAC (Acetadote®) is initiated with a 150 mg/kg loading dose infused over 60 minutes. This initial dose used to be administered over 15 minutes, although 60 minutes is now recommended to help alleviate any potential adverse, infusion-related reactions. After the loading dose is infused, a 50 mg/kg dose is then infused over 4 hours, followed by 100 mg/kg infused over 16 hours. This regimen results in a total dose of 300 mg/kg over 21 hours. As alluded to earlier, there are other regimens described in the literature. One such regimen consists of administering a loading dose of IV NAC of 140 mg/kg followed by 12 doses of 70 mg/kg every 4 hours.[4] It should be noted that no clear benefit exists between the two regimens; however, the one approved by the FDA is the 21-hour protocol.

Mucomyst® is an NAC product that is intended to be used for inhalation or oral administration. This product can be used for IV administration although it should only be used if Acetadote® is unavailable. When using Mucomyst® for IV administration, it is mixed and administered in the same way as Acetadote,® although an in-line 0.22 micron filter must be used during preparation.[8]

## Assessment

The case described depicts a scenario of severe hepatotoxicity associated with acetaminophen overdose and one in which conventional dosing with oral NAC would not be recommended for multiple reasons. The inability to assess the quantity of acetaminophen consumed or how much time had elapsed prior to admission direct the practitioner to the use of IV NAC. Additionally, the severity of poisoning in this patient appears to be very high. She was already encephalopathic, and her liver transaminase levels were well above any normal level. Rough estimates of the signs and symptoms of acetaminophen toxicity suggest that elevation in liver enzymes occur after 1 to 3 days of poisoning, with encephalopathy occurring upwards of 3 days after poisoning.[9] Even with rough estimates, this patient was well outside of the time frame in which conventional dosing of either oral or intravenous NAC has been administered with beneficial results. Further complicating the issue, she also consumed the acetaminophen with alcohol, a combination that can lead to increased hepatic damage.

Many of the cases seen at our institution are of a similar nature. Rarely can the acetaminophen overdose trauma patient be stratified according to existing nomograms because it is often difficult or impossible to assess the length of time that has elapsed since ingestion. In addition, many of these patients are admitted already showing signs of hepatotoxicity, if not hepatic failure. In these cases, a different strategy in dosing IV NAC is implemented.

Though not thoroughly described in the literature, the Illinois Poison Control Center recommends that "for patients with measurable acetaminophen levels and/or evidence of hepatotoxicity after completing entire treatment protocol, IV NAC should be continued at a rate of 100mg/kg in 1000 mL of 5% Dextrose (D$_5$W) over 16 hours until acetaminophen level is not detected and hepatotoxicity improves."[10] Although there are few data to support dosing IV NAC in the manner described in this case, professional opinion suggests that if there has been no early adverse reaction to IV NAC, continuing therapy in this manner is unlikely to be harmful.[11]

# Conclusion

Challenges in treating acetaminophen toxicity with NAC occur in those patients who cannot be stratified according to a nomogram and who present in the later stages of toxicity. As the severity of poisoning in a patient increases due to such factors as delayed time to NAC initiation or the concomitant consumption of alcohol or opioids, the thought of using oral NAC should shift towards using IV NAC. Numerous reports describe various dosing regimens of both oral and IV NAC, but none of these regimens have been shown to be superior. In addition, these studies focus on preventing hepatotoxicity and do not assess the patient who presents with hepatic failure. Despite the lack of data to support its benefit, recent literature recommends the use of continued NAC administration until there is firm evidence of improved hepatic function and states that the length of NAC administration should be determined by clinical improvement or outcome rather than by time or acetaminophen level.[12] Current policies written by the American College of Emergency Physicians have yet to make such a recommendation.[13]

Although it is difficult to recommend any treatment in which there are insufficient data to support its use, the way in which IV NAC was used in this case appears reasonable. Further studies comparing both IV to oral NAC while assessing duration of therapy are needed. Until that time, clinical and professional judgment should dictate treatment in cases of severe toxicity.

# References

1.  Kanter MZ. Comparison of oral and IV acetylcysteine in the treatment of acetaminophen poisoning. *Am J Health-Syst Pharm* 2006;63:1821-1827.
2.  Acetadote® Injection Product Information. Cumberland Pharmaceutical Inc, February 2006.
3.  Prescott LF. Oral or intravenous N-acetylcysteine for acetaminophen poisoning? *Ann Emerg Med* 2005;45:409-13.
4.  Smilkstein MJ, Bronstein AC, Linden C, et al. Acetaminophen overdose: A 48-hour intravenous n-acetylcysteine treatment protocol. *Ann Emerg Med* 1991;20(10):1058.
5.  Smilkstein, MJ, Knapp GL, Kulig KW, et al. Efficacy of oral N-acetylcysteine in the treatment of acetaminophen overdose. Analysis of the national multicenter study (1976-1975). *N Engl J Med* 1988;319:1557-62.
6.  Prescott LF, Illingworth RN, Critchley JA, et al. Intravenous N-acetylcysteine: the treatment of choice for paracetamol poisoning. *Br Med J* 1979;2:1097-100.
7.  Rumack BH, Matthew H: Acetaminophen poisoning and toxicity. Pediatrics1975; 5:871–876.
8.  Burda AM, Breier CJ, Wahl M. Illinois Poison Center: Nine facts about intravenous N-acetylcysteine in the setting of acetaminophen poisoning. ICHP KeePosted 2008: 34(3):22-24.
9.  Chyka PA. Clinical Toxicology. Pharmacotherapy, 4th Edition. Dipiro JT, et al., eds. Stamford, CT: Appleton and Lange; 1999;77-79.
10.  Illinois Poison Center. "Intravenous N-acetylcysteine therapy." Personal communication; Dec. 12, 2006.

11. Personal communication with Laurie Prescott, MD, FRCP, University of Edinburgh, Edinburgh, United Kingdom via email; Dec. 13, 2006.

12. Stravitz RT, Kramer AH, Davern T, et al. Intensive care of patients with acute liver failure: Recommendations of the U.S Acute Liver Failure Study Group. *Crit Care Med* 2007;35:2498-2508

13. Wolf SJ, Heard K, Sloan EP, et al. Clinical Policy: Critical issues in the management of patients presenting to the emergency department with acetaminophen overdose. *Ann Emerg Med* 2007;50(3):292-313.

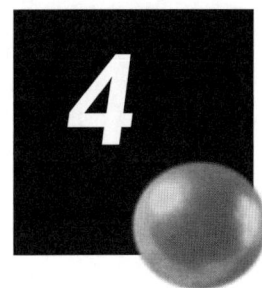

# Pharmacy Proofs: $Cl_{cr} \neq$ GFR

*Jaime L. Borkowski*

## Background and Introduction

In 1999, the National Kidney Foundation (NKF) organized the Kidney Disease Outcomes Quality Initiative (K/DOQI) to foster earlier identification of patients with kidney disease to help avoid progression of kidney disease and the development of end-stage renal disease (ESRD). K/DOQI clinical practice guidelines for chronic kidney disease evaluation and classification published in 2002 describe a new staging system for chronic kidney disease based on glomerular filtration rate (GFR). To promote more accurate determination of GFR, the guidelines also describe equations that the NKF considers appropriate to calculate an estimated GFR. The two equations identified for use in adults to determine GFR include the Cockcroft-Gault (C-G) equation and the Modification of Diet in Renal Disease (MDRD) equation. These guidelines noted that the MDRD equation performs better in estimating the GFR compared with the C-G equation.[1]

An effort by the National Kidney Disease Education Program (NKDEP) to standardize serum creatinine values lead to an increased exposure of practitioners to the MDRD equation. In 2006, the NKDEP formed a laboratory working group to discuss issues related to creatinine standardization. It was recommended that Isotope Dilution Mass Spectometry (IDMS) be designated as the gold standard for creatinine assays, and assay manufacturers recalibrate routine serum creatinine methods to be traceable to an IDMS standard. The new serum creatinine standardization results in a new normal range for serum creatinine that is lower than the range with traditional assays. The standardization of the assays allows for a more accurate calculation of GFR using the MDRD equation. It was also recommended that GFR based on MDRD be automatically reported whenever a serum creatinine is reported for adults.[2]

With the widespread availability of the GFR based on the MDRD equation that has resulted from these efforts, questions arise frequently regarding the clinical applications of the GFR compared with those of the creatinine clearance ($Cl_{cr}$) as calculated by the C-G equation. Does the GFR represent the $Cl_{cr}$ and can they be used interchangeably? If the MDRD equation is considered a more accurate estimate of GFR, shouldn't that be used instead of the C-G when determining renal function for all purposes, including renal dose adjustments?

# Cockcroft-Gault Equation

The original study that derived the C-G equation was published in 1976.[3] It was based on a group of 534 primarily male inpatients. The patients ranged in age from 18 to 92 years, and their measured $Cl_{cr}$ levels ranged from 11 mL/min to normal. The measured $Cl_{cr}$ was determined by 24-hour urine collections in each patient, and at least two collections were performed on each subject to assess stability of renal function. The newly derived equation was compared with three published equations (Jelliffe I and II, Edwards, and Whyte) and the Siersbaek-Nielsen nomogram. The test group of patients consisted of a subset of the total population of 236 men that had two measured $Cl_{cr}$ within 20% of each other, 24-hour creatinine excretion >10 mg/kg, and adequate records.

The investigators found that of all the methods to estimate renal function, the new equation (what we now know as the C-G equation) and the Siersbaek-Nielsen Nomogram had the best correlation coefficients between measured and estimated $Cl_{cr}$ (r = 0.83 and 0.84, respectively). The correlation coefficients for the other three equations tested ranged from 0.73-0.80.[3]

The C-G equation originally published is as follows:

$$Cl_{cr} \text{ (mL/min)} = \frac{[140 - \text{Age (years)}] \times \text{Weight (kg)}}{72 \times S_{Cr}} \times 0.85 \text{ (for females)}$$

The original study used actual body weight in the equation, however, the authors stated that the use of an ideal body weight (IBW) may be necessary in patients with marked obesity or ascites instead of actual body weight to obtain a more accurate estimation of $Cl_{cr}$.[3] It is common practice to use the ideal body weight or adjusted body weight in clinical practice for drug dosing at this time.

# Limitations and Uses of Cockcroft-Gault

Although it is widely used due to its ease of use in clinical practice, the C-G equation has many limitations. One of the most important limitations is that the use of urine creatinine as the standard on which the equation was derived creates an inherent problem with using the result to estimate GFR. Although creatinine is filtered through the glomerulus, it is also secreted by the proximal tubule into the urine. Creatinine in the urine, therefore, overestimates the clearance by the glomerulus (due to the extra creatinine in the urine from this secretion by the proximal tubule).[1] Because the C-G equation was derived based on the 24-hour urine creatinine measurement, the equation automatically predicts a result that is slightly greater than the actual GFR. This result is the $Cl_{cr}$ and cannot be considered synonymous to the GFR because of this fact.

Another limitation of the C-G equation is that it was not originally studied in many females. Ninety-six percent of the original population was male. The $Cl_{cr}$ is only applicable when the patient's renal function is at steady state, as well. Finally, the body surface area (BSA) of the patients was not taken into account, and the results of the equation are significantly affected by muscle mass.[3]

Because of the ease of use in clinical practice, the renal function as calculated by C-G has been applied to many clinical situations. Examples of uses of the C-G equation include detection of the onset of renal insufficiency, adjustment of medications excreted by the kidneys, evaluation of the effectiveness of therapy for progressive renal disease, and documentation of eligibility for reimbursement from programs such as the Medicare End-Stage Renal Disease Program.[4]

## Modification of Diet in Renal Disease Study

The original MDRD study was not performed to determine a new equation to predict renal function. Published in 1994 by Klahr et al., it was actually designed to determine the effects of dietary protein restriction and blood pressure control on the progression of renal disease.[5] Patients who were included in the study were 18-70 years of age, had a serum creatinine ($S_{Cr}$) of 1.2-7 mg/dL (females) or 1.4-7mg/dL (males) or a GFR < 70 mL/min/1.73m$^2$, and a mean arterial pressure of ≤ 125 mm Hg. Patients were excluded if they were pregnant, weighed < 80% or >160% of their IBW, had diabetes mellitus requiring insulin therapy, urinary protein >10 g/day, a history of renal transplant, chronic medical conditions, or there were doubts about their potential compliance with the study parameters. The patient population of the study is particularly important to note because this is the patient population that was used by Levey in 1999 to derive some new equations to predict GFR.

For the purposes of their study, Levey used the data for 1628 of the 1785 patients who were originally entered into the baseline period of the MDRD and had GFR data and other variables that they intended to consider for inclusion in the new model.[4] The MDRD study determined a reference GFR by measuring the renal clearance of $^{125}$I-iothalamate, and a reference $Cl_{cr}$ was determined using a 24-hour urine collection. The investigators used multiple regression to evaluate multiple variables and to determine which ones significantly affected GFR. Some patients were used as a training sample in which the coefficients for each variable were determined. The remaining patients made up the validation sample in which the models were tested for accuracy.

Interestingly, the mean measured GFR among the patients in the MDRD study was 39.8 mL/min/1.73m$^2$, whereas the mean measured Clcr was 48.6 mL/min/1.73m$^2$. These findings demonstrate the principle that $Cl_{cr}$ overestimates actual GFR. The $Cl_{cr}$ as estimated by C-G overestimated the actual GFR by about 16%. This is actually not a large difference when considering the low values one is dealing with for GFR.[4]

The two equations (equations "6" and "7") derived in the MDRD equation study resulted in the lowest variability in predicted GFR compared to measured GFR ($R^2$ = 91.2% and 90.3%, respectively). The main difference between the two equations is that Equation 6 included variables relating to urine chemistry, while equation 7 excluded the urine chemistry values. The median absolute error for C-G was 6.8 mL/min/1.73m$^2$ compared to that for MDRD of 3.8 mL/min/1.73m$^2$ (without adjustment for bias). The authors concluded that the MDRD equations 6 and 7 are more accurate than C-G in estimating actual GFR (see Equation #1 below).[4]

A year after the MDRD equation was published, the authors worked with NKDEP to develop an equation that was easier to use in clinical practice than the 6-variable equation described in the first study. The abbreviated MDRD equation, or MDRD-4 equation, excludes the use of serum urea nitrogen (SUN) and albumin in the calculation of GFR. The authors found that there was still a good correlation with actual GFR with the MDRD 4 study (see Equation #2 below).[6]

The following are the most commonly used versions of the MDRD equation:

1)   MDRD Equation #7 [4]

GFR (mL/min/1.73m$^2$) = 170 × P$_{cr}^{-0.999}$ × Age$^{-0.176}$ × 0.762 if female × 1.180 if black × SUN$^{-0.170}$ × Alb$^{+0.318}$

2)   MDRD Abbreviated Version (4-Variable) [6]

GFR (mL/min/1.73m$^2$) = 186 × S$_{Cr}^{-1.154}$ × age$^{-0.203}$ × (0.742 if female) × (1.210 if black)

3)   IDMS-traceable MDRD [7]

GFR (mL/min/1.73m$^2$) = 175 × S$_{Cr}^{-1.154}$ × age$^{-0.203}$ × (0.742 if female) × (1.212 if black)

The third equation listed is a version of the abbreviated MDRD equation that was derived to be used with the new serum creatinine (S$_{Cr}$) range that resulted from the standardization of serum creatinine assays to an IDMS-traceable standard described previously. The coefficients for this equation have been adjusted slightly, although the variables are all the same: SCr, age, gender, and ethnicity.[7]

## Limitations of MDRD

The main limitations of the GFR as calculated by the MDRD equation are related to the patient populations in which the equation was tested (or not tested). The groups in which the MDRD equation has not been adequately validated include patients without renal disease, people <18 years old or >70 years old, pregnant women, ethnicities other than Caucasian or Black, patients with serious comorbid conditions, and patients with low creatinine generation.[4] As with the Cockcroft-Gault equation and many other equations used to estimate renal function, the MDRD equation is not accurate when the patient's renal function is not at steady state. Finally, according to the authors, if the GFR is being used to adjust the doses of renally cleared medications, the result must be unadjusted for BSA (converted from mL/min/1.73m$^2$ to mL/min).

## Comparison of C-G and MDRD for Drug Adjustments

Wargo et al.[8] conducted an observational analysis of 409 inpatients to assess the effects of the C-G equation versus the MDRD equation in determining the need for dosage adjustments in eight common antimicrobials at their institution. They included patients with S$_{Cr}$ of 1.3-3.0 mg/dL and documented chronic kidney disease (CKD) of stages 3-5. They excluded patients with acute renal failure, ESRD on dialysis, CKD stages 1 or 2, and race other than Caucasian or Black. In the study, the investigators compared what dosing adjustments would be needed based on both the C-G and MDRD equations. They found an overall discordant rate of 20-36% between the recommended dose adjustments for each equation (p < 0.001). Antimicrobials would have been dosed differently about 25% of the time depending on which equation was used. The majority of the discordance existed when the manufacturer recommended adjustment based on C-G, but adjustment was not required based on MDRD.

Gill et al.[9] performed a similar study that was a retrospective, cross-sectional study of 180 elderly patients in long-term care facilities. The population included patients with a mean age of 85 years, 78% of whom were female, 68% of whom were white, and 30% of whom were Asian. This population was different from the original MDRD population due to the higher average age and the subpopulation of Asian patients, both groups that the MDRD equation has not been well-validated in. They evaluated the effects of the respective equations on dosing adjustments for amantadine and digoxin. The study found a slightly higher rate of discordance in dosing between the two equations in the Asian patients, but this result was non-significant (p = 0.16). Reductions in the dose of amantadine would have been required in 70.0% of patients based on the MDRD equation and in 91.1% of patients based on C-G. Reductions of the digoxin dose would have been required in 25.7% of patients based on MDRD and in 58.1% of patients based on C-G.

These studies demonstrate that the dosing recommendations for many medications are clearly not the same when using C-G versus MDRD to determine renal function. The studies did not determine the patients' actual GFR using a gold-standard test such as the renal clearance of $^{125}$I-iothalamate, but they instead attempted to assess the effects of each equation on what would be done with the medication dose in clinical practice.

## National Organization Recommendations Relating to Drug Dosing

The U.S. Food and Drug Administration (FDA) published the most recent Guidance for Industry document regarding study design to determine pharmacokinetics in patients with impaired renal function in May of 1998.[10] This document includes recommendations on how to determine renal function for studying drugs that are renally cleared. Creatinine clearance is specified in this document as a commonly used method of determining renal function for patients in studies, and the document also specifies the C-G equation as an acceptable way to calculate the $Cl_{cr}$. The document goes further in noting that other measures of renal function can be used to provide additional understanding of the effect of renal impairment on the kinetics of the drug, but these other measures should not be considered for use as alternatives to the more commonly used method such as $Cl_{cr}$. The guidance document was published prior to the MDRD study, so it did not take the MDRD equation into consideration. Drug manufacturers continue to use $Cl_{cr}$ as calculated by C-G as the primary method of determining renal function in patients in their drug studies, however, and therefore are making their dosing recommendations based on this value. Attempts to contact the FDA to inquire as to whether new recommendations that address the use of MDRD in drug studies are being developed were unsuccessful.

The Laboratory Working Group formed by NKDEP to address creatinine assay standardization also addressed the issue of which equation to use when dosing medications that are renally cleared. In their Recommendations for Pharmacists and Authorized Drug Prescribers,[11] the working group specifically notes the lack of equivalence between the $Cl_{cr}$ as calculated by C-G and the GFR as calculated by MDRD. They recommend that practitioners continue to use dose adjustments based on recommendations from manufacturers for specific drugs as approved by the FDA.

## Uses of MDRD GFR

Based on the limitations of the GFR as calculated by the MDRD equation, the uses one may see this result used for in practice include early detection renal dysfunction, assessment of disease progression and prognosis, evaluation of treatment, and defining the need for dialysis or transplantation.[12] Use of the MDRD GFR for dosing of medications is not recommended at this time.

# Effects of Creatinine Standardization on Clinical Practice

As noted previously, the NKDEP has promoted a nationwide standardization of creatinine assays that results in a lower normal range for $S_{Cr}$ values. This affects the $Cl_{cr}$ result obtained when using the C-G calculation. The new $S_{Cr}$ values have been estimated to be anywhere from 5-20% lower than the values determined using the previous creatinine assays.[13] This will result in falsely elevated estimations of renal function. It probably affects more patients in those groups on the cusp of two different doses; however, it is a factor that practitioners need to take into consideration. This makes other patient factors even more important to consider, including the trend in the $S_{Cr}$, patient clinical status, type of drug being dosed, and potential risks to the patient of over- or underdosing.

# Conclusion

The differences between the C-G $Cl_{cr}$ and the MDRD GFR will not affect a large number of patients, especially if the practitioner is converting the GFR to mL/min before using for dosage adjustments. However, the C-G $Cl_{cr}$ should continue to be used for drug dose adjustments at this time. The standardization of creatinine assays is causing the $S_{Cr}$ results to be about 5-20% lower than previous values so taking this into consideration along with other important patient-specific factors is extremely important when evaluating the need to adjust a medication dose based on renal function.

# References

1. National Kidney Foundation. K/DOQI clinical practice guidelines for chronic kidney disease: evaluation, classification, and stratification. Kidney Disease Outcome Quality Initiative. *Am J Kidney Dis* 2002; 2 Suppl 1:S1-S266.
2. Myers GL, Miller G, Coresh J, et al. Recommendations for improving serum creatinine measurement: a report from the Laboratory Working Group of the National Kidney Disease Education Program. *Clin Chem* 2006;52(1):5-18.
3. Cockcroft DW, Gault MH. Prediction of creatinine clearance from serum creatinine. *Nephron* 1976;16:31-41.
4. Levey AS, Bosch JP, Lewis JB, et al. A more accurate method to estimate glomerular filtration rate from serum creatinine: a new prediction equation. *Ann Intern Med* 1999;130(6):461-70.

5. Klahr S, et al. The effects of dietary protein restriction and blood-pressure control on the progression of chronic renal disease. *N Engl J Med* 1994;330:877-84.

6. Levey AS, et al. A simplified equation to predict glomerular filtration rate from serum creatinine [Abstract]. *J Am Soc Nephrol* 2000;11:155A.

7. Levey AS, et al. Using standardized serum creatinine values in the modification of diet in renal disease study equation for estimating glomerular filtration rate. *Ann Intern Med* 2006;145(4):247-54.

8. Wargo KA, et al. Comparison of the Modification of Diet in Renal Disease and Cockcroft-Gault equations for antimicrobial dosage adjustments. *Ann Pharmacother* 2006;40:1248-53.

9. Gill J, et al. Use of GFR equations to adjust drug doses in an elderly multi-ethnic group—a cautionary tale. *Nephrol Dial Transplant* 2007;22:2894-2899.

10. Guidance for Industry: Pharmacokinetics in patients with impaired renal function—study design, data analysis, and impact on dosing and labeling. U.S. Department of Health and Human Services Food and Drug Administration; May 1998. Accessed at http://www.fda.gov/cder/guidance/1449fnl.pdf on 2/9/08.

11. Creatinine Standardization Program—Recommendations for Pharmacists and Authorized Drug Prescribers. NKDEP, July 2006. Accessed at http://www.nkdep.nih.gov/labprofessionals/Pharm_Recommendations_508.pdf on 2/9/08.

12. Prigent A. Monitoring renal function and limitations of renal function tests. *Semin Nucl Med* 2008;38:32-46.

13. Wade W, Spruill W. New serum creatinine assay standardization: implications for drug dosing. *Ann Pharmacother* 2007;41:475-80.

# 5

# Succinylcholine in the Critically Ill Patient: When Is It Not OK+?

*Clyde Birringer*

## Hospital

Meriter Hospital is a 448-bed non-profit community hospital located in Madison, Wisconsin. Meriter provides comprehensive health services for residents of southern Wisconsin and areas of northwest Illinois and is a major teaching affiliate of the University of Wisconsin. It is the fifth largest hospital in Wisconsin.

## Background

The Intensive Care Units (ICU) at Meriter use many high risk drugs in daily practice. Efforts have been made to improve the safe use of these high risk drugs at our hospital. One example of a high risk drug causing a severe adverse effect in our ICU is succinylcholine induced hyperkalemia in a patient with disuse atrophy. Since little was known about the risk of hyperkalemia in this patient subset, a literature review was performed and a summary given to our physicians.

## Challenges

Neuromuscular blocking agents (NMBA) are high risk drugs used in critically ill patients when short term paralysis is necessary. This can include procedures such as endotracheal intubation or EEG testing. The choice of NMBA is often based on onset and duration of action, mode of elimination, disease and drug interactions and potential adverse effects. Neuromuscular blocking agents are often used prior to endotracheal intubation, EEG testing, or other tests that require the patient to lie flaccid and still. Because of this, some critically ill patients may require short-term paralysis during their hospital stay. Succinyl-choline is the only marketed *depolarizing* neuromuscular blocking agent and is commonly used because of its fast onset (< 1 min) and short duration (~5 - 10 minutes).[1]

Succinylcholine is associated with a number of serious or life-threatening adverse effects. These include the following:[1]

- Apnea: This is a direct result of the neuromuscular blocking activity of the drug on the diaphragm and other muscles of the respiratory tree.
- Bradycardia: This effect is likely due to increase in vagal tone through cholinergic receptor stimulation in the myocardium.
- Malignant hyperthermia: This reaction occurs in genetically predisposed patients as a result of hypermetabolism of skeletal muscles.
- Increased intracranial pressure: Contractions of extraocular muscles may transiently increase ICP by ~ 8 mmHg for up to 10 minutes in patients receiving the drug.
- Hyperkalemia: Depolarization of acetylcholine receptors at neuromuscular junction results in release of potassium from muscle and increased potassium concentrations (0.5–1 mEq/L) in most individuals. This occurs within minutes after administration of succinylcholine. Patients with certain pathological states or interactions may experience profound hyperkalemia and death following the administration of succinylcholine.

## Review

With certain pathological states or conditions, up-regulation of acetylcholine receptors occurs in the muscle. These receptors can spread and occupy all of the muscle membrane. Following stimulation of these sensitive receptors with succinylcholine, large amounts of potassium are released from the muscle membrane. Pathologic conditions that increase the risk of hyperkalemia with succinylcholine include the following[2]:

- Upper or lower motor defect
  - Spinal cord injury
  - Peripheral nerve injury or neuropathy
  - Parkinson's disease
  - Muscular dystrophy
  - Multiple sclerosis
  - Paraplegia/ hemiplegia
- Burns/thermal injury
- Severe infection
- Prolonged chemical denervation
  - Muscle relaxants (including non-depolarizing neuromuscular blocking agents)
  - Magnesium
  - Tetanus
- *Disuse Atrophy or Immobilization*

Many of these conditions that predispose patients to hyperkalemia have been well documented over the years.[2,3,4] Recently, much of the interest is focused on the role that immobilization or disuse atrophy alone may play. Within the first few days of immobilization, muscle atrophy and upregulation of acetylcholine receptors occurs. In patients with pathological states, hyperkalemia has been reported after administering succinylcholine in as little as 4 days[2]. It is not known how long it takes for patients to be at risk from succinylcholine-induced hyperkalemia with immobility alone. Some clinicians recommend avoiding this drug in patients who are immobile for as little as 2 to 3 days or in patients with pathologic states that put them at risk.[2]

## Diagnosis

Hyperkalemia is usually diagnosed with laboratory testing with potassium levels between 5.1 mEq/L to 6.0 mEq/L reflecting mild hyperkalemia, 6.1 mEq/L to 7.0 mEq/L, moderate hyperkalemia, and levels above 7 mEq/L, severe hyperkalemia. Life threatening arrhythmias can occur, especially with Potassium levels > 7 mEq/L. In most patients without risk factors, Potassium levels will generally increase by 0.5 – 1 mEq/L following succinylcholine.[1]: Potassiums levels more than 7 mEq/L have been reported after administering succinylcholine in patients who are at risk[2,3,4]:. Hyperkalemia can also be diagnosed with an ECG. Figure 5.1 shows an ECG that indicates hyperkalemia with spiked T waves, loss of P waves, and wide QRS in a

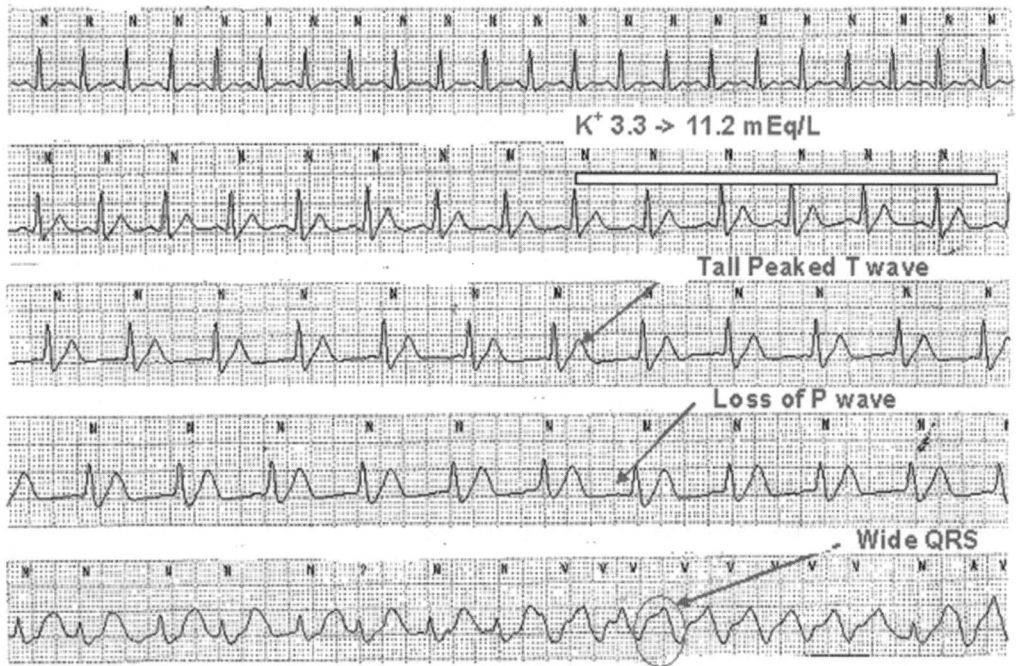

**Figure 5.1.** ECG that indicates hyperkalemia with spiked T waves, loss of P waves, and wide QRS in a patient who had no known risk factors other than immobility for 21 days and who received succinylcholine minutes earlier.

patient who had no known risk factors other than immobility for 21 days and who received succinylcholine minutes earlier.

## Prevention

Screening patients for predisposing pathologic states and conditions before administering succinylcholine or using alternative agents can prevent succinylcholine-induced hyperkalemia. Suggested alternative agents include the following:

- Anesthetic drugs, such as propofol or etomidate, which can be used for tracheal intubation when an anesthesiologist is available.
- A fast onset, short-acting nondepolarizing neuromuscular blocking agent, such as rocuronium (Zemuron®), which does not cause hyperkalemia. Doses in the range of 0.9 – 1.2 mg/kg IV push will usually result in sufficient paralysis in 1 – 2 minutes and last 60 to 90 minutes.

## Conclusion

Succinylcholine is associated with a number of serious and life-threatening adverse effects, including hyperkalemia. The risk of these adverse effects can be minimized with knowledge and understanding of the underlying causes and the patient populations at risk. Pharmacists can play a key role in recommending safer agents when necessary.

## References

1. QUELICIN(R) IV injection, Product information: succinylcholine chloride IV injection. Hospira, Inc., Lake Forest, IL, 2005.
2. Jeevendra Martyn JA, Richtsfeld M. Succinylcholine-induced hyperkalemia in acquired pathologic states. *Anesthesiology* 2006;104:158-169.
3. Huggins RM, Kennedy WK, Melroy MJ, et al. Cardiac arrest from succinylcholine-induced hyperkalemia. *Am J Health-System Pharm* 2003;60:693-697.
4. Allen ME. Succinylcholine-induced cardiac arrest in a patient with no known risk factors. *Crit Care Med* 2006;34:A162.

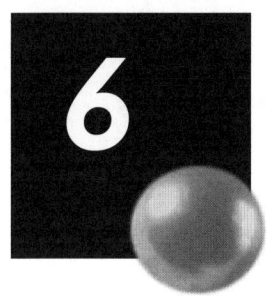

# 6

# Insulin Sliding Scales: To Use or Not to Use, That Is the Question

*Jon Horton*

The origins of sliding scale insulin can be traced back to Elliott Joslin, who recommended its use not to manage hyperglycemia but rather control glucosuria.[1] Insulin dosing was guided by colorimetric results derived from testing urine for the presence of varying concentrations of glucose. Despite availability of blood glucose testing in the hospital setting,[2] it was not until the introduction of capillary blood glucose monitoring in the 1980s, that the first modification of the urine glucose algorithms occurred, incorporating the use of capillary blood glucose targets.[3-5] Subsequently, this practice has been widely applied to the routine monitoring of patients with diabetes as well as patients with stress-related hyperglycemia.

The use of sliding scale insulin in the management of hospitalized patients is deeply embedded in the medical culture secondary to convenience, simplicity, and promptness of treatment.[6] Despite these significant advantages, this treatment modality has been criticized by many because it is a reactive rather than a proactive treatment for avoiding the development of hyperglycemia. Also, it depends upon the incorrect assumption that insulin sensitivity is uniform among patients and lacks prospective, randomized, controlled clinical trials that demonstrate improved glycemic control through its use.[7] It has also been suggested that this "reactive" approach can lead to rapid changes in blood glucose levels, exacerbating both hyperglycemia and hypoglycemia.[7-9]

## Impact of Hyperglycemia in Hospitalized Patients

The macro and micro vascular long-term complications of hyperglycemia are well known,[10] but it has only more recently been demonstrated that hyperglycemia in hospitalized patients also has a significant influence on hospital stay, disability, and death.[11] Umpierrez et al. demonstrated that when comparing patients who were normoglycemic, patients with a new onset hyperglycemia had increased average hospital stays, increased admission rates to the intensive care unit, increased transfer rates to transitional care units, increased admissions to nursing home facilities, decreased discharge rates to home and an 18 fold increase in mortality.[11] In addition, diabetic patients experiencing hyperglycemia had a 2.5 fold increase in mortality when compared to hospitalized diabetics with normoglycemia.[11] Pomposelli et al. demonstrated that postoperative day 1 hyperglycemia (glucose levels greater than 220 mg/dL) is a sensitive predictor of nosocomial infection.[12] Data continues to become available demonstrating that the presence of hyperglycemia, not only in those patients with the diagnosis of diabetes, but also those patients who are not known diabetics is important in hospitalized patients.

## Causes of Hyperglycemia in Hospitalized Patients

Hospitalized patients suffer metabolic stress responses related to increases in stress hormones and peptides responsible for increasing glucose concentrations and or decreasing insulin secretion.[9] The presence of hyperglycemia is known to cause immune dysfunction, which ultimately increases the dissemination of infection. Glucose and insulin dysregulation increases free fatty acid (FFA) metabolism, resulting in the increased formation of reactive oxygen species. FFA

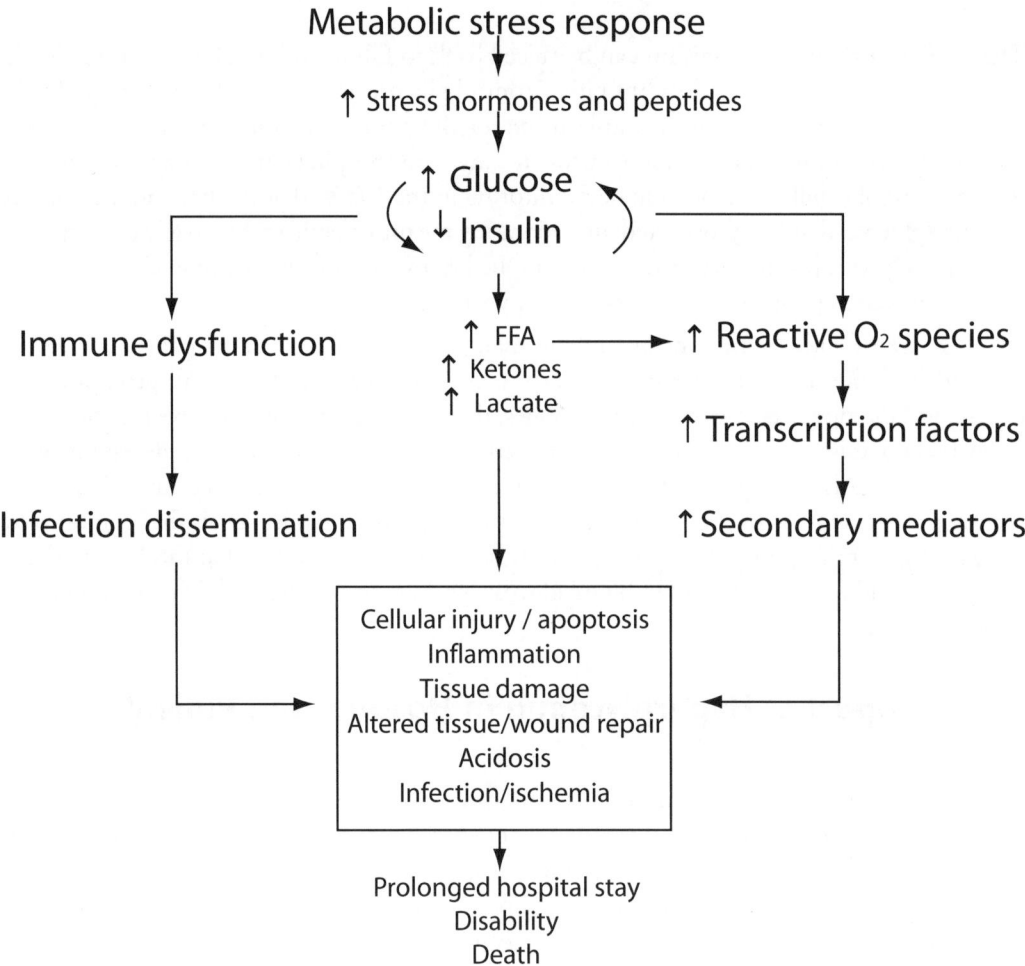

**Figure 6.1.** Link between hyperglycemia and poor hospital outcomes. Hyperglycemia and relative insulin deficiency caused by metabolic stress triggers immune dysfunction, release of fuel substrates, and other mediators such as ROS. Tissue and organ injury occur via the combined insults of infection, direct fuel-mediated injury, oxidative stress and other downstream mediators. Reprinted with permission from Clement S, Braithwaite SS, Magee MF, et al. Management of diabetes and hyperglycemia in hospitals. *Diabetes Care* 2004; 27:553-597.

metabolism is also responsible for ketone and lactate production. Complications related to all of these effects ultimately result in cellular injury/apoptosis, inflammation, tissue damage, altered tissue/wound repair, acidosis, thrombosis, and infarction/ischemia (Fig. 6.1).[9]

Based upon the potential for complications, it is recommended that hospitalized patients be evaluated for the presence of hyperglycemia. Fasting blood glucose values greater than 126 mg/dL or a random blood glucose greater than 200 mg/dL are appropriate indicators for the need of additional evaluation and treatment. Based upon the American College of Endocrinology Position Statement on Inpatient Diabetes and Metabolic Control, goals for hospitalized patients include: preprandial blood glucose less than 110 mg/dL (6.1 mmol/L) or postprandial blood glucose less than 180 mg/dL (10 mmol/L).[13]

## Pitfalls of Sliding Scale Insulin

Once hyperglycemia is identified, the most effective treatment strategy includes the utilization of insulin therapy.[13] Unfortunately, sliding scale insulin, which has been described as being ineffective, is used almost reflexively as the insulin strategy in the hospital setting.[7]

As previously described there are numerous reasons for the ineffectiveness of sliding scale insulin therapy. Queale et al.[14] demonstrated that sliding scale schedules written on admission often remain unchanged throughout a patient's hospital stay despite the presence of hyperglycemia. These findings are supported by more recent studies that demonstrate that despite persistently elevated blood glucose levels, adjustments in timing or the dose of insulin were made infrequently with no adjustments being made in 81% of patients.[15] Although many hospitals have promoted the use of standardized sliding scales to avoid medication errors, such standardization does not allow for the normal variance in patient to patient sensitivity to the glucose lowering effects of insulin.

Umpierrez et al. demonstrated in a randomized controlled trial that a protocol utilizing intensification of a sliding scale regimen based upon a patient's responsiveness to insulin was able to achieve glycemic targets in approximately 40% of patients.[16] Failure to intensify insulin dosing appears to be a significant barrier to glycemic control and may explain why earlier studies were unable to identify a treatment effect from sliding scale therapy. Matheny et al.[17] in a retrospective analysis of non-intensive care unit patients with diabetes, demonstrated that patients received treatment intensification for only 22% of the days when hyperglycemia was present. This data also showed that intensification of scheduled and sliding scale insulin, but not oral medications were associated with reductions in average daily glucose. Matheny's data, demonstrating improvement in glycemic control even in the absence of a treatment regimen, emphasizes the importance of the patient's overall clinical status and severity of illness on glucose management.[17]

## Recommended Management of Hyperglycemia in Hospitalized Patients

Once hospitalized, diabetic patients often have oral hypoglycemic agents held secondary to concerns over dietary intake and the need to withhold meals prior to diagnostic procedures and interventions. A conservative treatment strategy should include withholding oral agents and the use of sliding scale insulin with intensification of therapy based upon the patient's degree

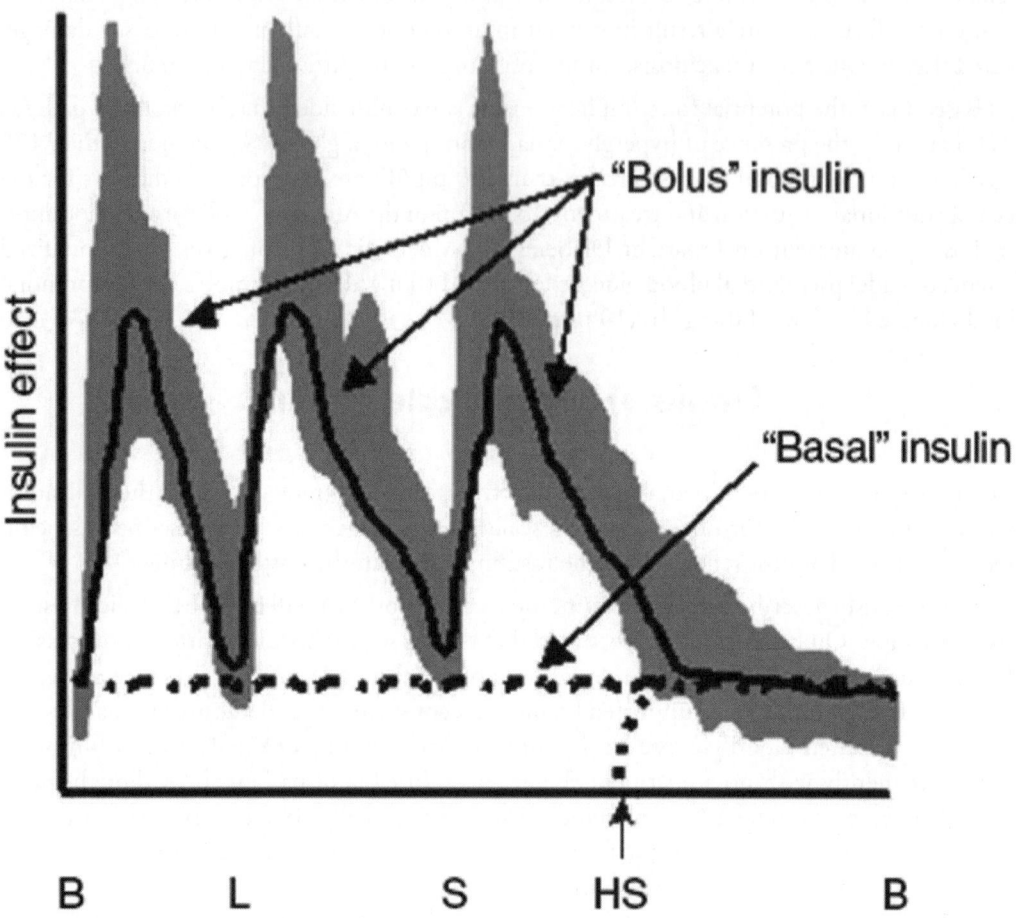

**Figure 6.2.** Schematic demonstrating basal and bolus concept for restoring insulin secretory profiles. This figure depicts, in the shaded area, the normal insulin action. Multiple daily analog injections mimic well the physiologic profile by providing prandial insulin coverage, i.e., "bolus" insulin. "Basal" insulin replacement controls the nocturnal, fasting, and postabsorptive periods. Reprinted with permission from Cefalu WT. *Pharmacotherapy for the Treatment of Patients with Type 2 Diabetes Mellitus: Rationale and Specific Agents. Clin Pharmacol Therap* 2007; 81:636-649.

of hyperglycemia. Unfortunately, based upon all data available, this alternative will likely not prove to be adequate therapy for the majority of patients.

Once a patient has been identified as being hyperglycemic, a hospitalized patient's insulin regimen must be actively managed to achieve glucose goals. Umpierrez et al. demonstrated implementation of a basal bolus strategy in patients with type 2 diabetes (Fig. 6.2) which resulted in targeted glucose levels in the majority of patients when compared with patients receiving only intensification of sliding scale insulin therapy.[16] Additionally, data from the RABBIT 2 trial demonstrates the effectiveness of a basal bolus insulin dosing strategy in managing hyperglycemia in patients who failed initial management of sliding scale therapy ( Fig. 6.3).[16]

# Managing a Basal Bolus Insulin Regimen in Hospitalized Diabetic Patients

The first step in providing normoglycemia is identifying an appropriate insulin regimen after careful evaluation of a patient's medical history and degree of hyperglycemia. Umpierrez in the RABBIT 2 Trial[16] evaluated a basal bolus protocol for the management of hospitalized type 2 diabetic patients in comparison to an intensified sliding scale and demonstrated value of basal insulin in combination with meal related doses in avoiding hyperglycemia.

The treatment protocol included discontinuation of oral agents and calculation of a total daily insulin dose of 0.4 units per kilogram for patients with blood glucose concentrations between 140 and 200 mg/dL or 0.5 units per kilogram for patients with blood glucoses between 201 and 400 mg/dL. According to the RABBIT 2 Trial, 50% of the total daily dose of insulin should be provided in the form of basal insulin and the other half of the total daily dose of

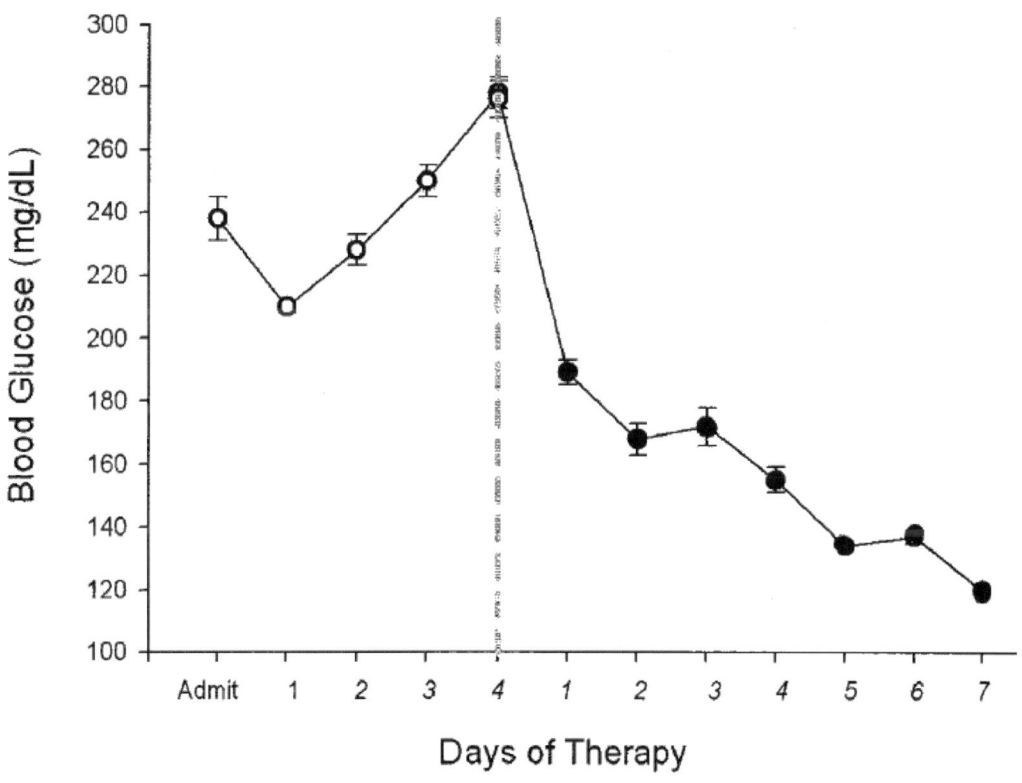

**Figure 6.3.** Mean blood glucose concentration in subjects who remained with severe hyperglycemia despite increasing doses of regular insulin per the sliding-scale protocol (open circles). Glycemic control rapidly improved after switching to the basal-bolus insulin regimen (closed circles). P < 0.05. Reprinted with permission from Umpierrez GE, Palacio A, Smiley D. Randomized study of basal-bolus insulin therapy in the inpatient management of patients with type 2 diabetes (RABBIT 2 Trial). *Diabetes Care* 2007; 30:2181-2185.

insulin is administered in three equally divided doses before each meal as a rapid acting insulin analog.[16] Point-of-care glucoses were measured routinely based upon a patient's dietary status and correctional doses of a rapid-acting insulin analog were administered as described.

## Basal Insulin Dosing Titration

Patients unable to eat or who had meals held, received long-acting insulin doses, but had scheduled preprandial doses of rapid-acting insulin withheld. Intensification of the basal dosage regimen was achieved by increasing the basal insulin dose by 20% when fasting; preprandial glucose levels were greater than 140 mg/dL. Conversely, the basal dose of insulin was decreased by 20% after an episode of hypoglycemia (defined as blood glucose less than 70 mg/dL). This study protocol, with intensification of insulin dosing regimen, successfully achieved glycemic control in approximately 70% of patients.

## Correctional Dosing

Correctional dosing refers to the provision of supplemental insulin to correct point-of-care results and reduce glucose levels. Correctional or supplemental doses of insulin are in their most simplistic form, a sliding scale, but they are given in addition to regularly scheduled meal related doses. In the RABBIT 2 Trial, an "insulin sensitive" sliding scale was administered every 6 hours (6-12-6-12) for patients who were not able to eat and a "usual" correctional scale was administered before meals and at bedtime for patients who were eating (Fig. 6.4).[16] The use of correctional insulin when given preprandially will help correct postprandial glucose levels.

| | ☐ Insulin sensitive | ☐ Usual |
|---|---|---|
| Blood glucose (mg/dl) | | |
| >141–180 | 2 | 4 |
| 181–220 | 4 | 6 |
| 221–260 | 6 | 8 |
| 261–300 | 8 | 10 |
| 301–350 | 10 | 12 |
| 351–400 | 12 | 14 |
| >400 | 14 | 16 |

**Figure 6.4.** Correctional or supplemental scales utilized in patients who were unable to eat were administered according to the "insulin sensitive" column every 6 hours and patients who were eating were administered before meals and before bedtime according to the "usual" column. For patients who were eating, these doses were given in addition to regularly scheduled preprandial doses. Reprinted with permission from Umpierrez GE, Palacio A, Smiley D. Randomized study of basal-bolus insulin therapy in the inpatient management of patients with type 2 diabetes (RABBIT 2 Trial). *Diabetes Care* 2007; 30:2181-2185.

# Stress-Related Hyperglycemia

In the landmark observational trial by Umpierrez et al.[11] one third of all patients who developed hyperglycemia during their hospitalization were patients in whom a prior diagnosis of diabetes was absent. These patients represent either undiagnosed type 2 diabetics or patients who are suffering from stress related hyperglycemia. The absence of a diabetes diagnosis is not protective in this patient population. Umpierrez demonstrated that the presence of hyperglycemia in undiagnosed patients is associated with significant morbidity and mortality.[11] Unfortunately, the majority of patients with hyperglycemia are not treated. Despite "new onset hyperglycemia" at admission, Umpierrez showed that only 13% of patients received orders for a change to a diabetic diet; 2% were initiated on oral hypoglycemic agents; 6% received scheduled insulin regimens; and 35% received sliding-scale insulin.[11]

Evaluation and diagnosis of diabetes may be helpful in targeting drug therapy. Patients who are diagnosed with diabetes can be treated successfully as outlined in the RABBIT 2 Trial. Little data is available to suggest a treatment protocol for the management of hyperglycemia in non-diabetic patients. The principles of insulin management as outlined by the RABBIT 2 Trial may prove beneficial in managing hyperglycemia in this patient population.

# Conclusion

Achieving glycemic control in more patients may require evaluation of outpatient therapy. In addition to considering current glucose values, it may be necessary to consider alteration of treatment based upon a patient's degree of glycemic control prior to admission. Likewise, the contribution of postprandial hyperglycemia on morbidity and mortality has yet to be elucidated. Additional or tighter control might be gained by evaluating postprandial glucose excursions (values greater than 180mg/dL).[13] To improve postprandial control, correctional doses of insulin may need to be administered 2 hours postprandially. Subsequent titration of preprandial insulin doses should be undertaken to improve glycemic control after meals until postprandial glycemic goals are achieved.

Reductions of complications associated with hyperglycemia may be achieved by implementing standardized subcutaneous insulin order sets that promote the use of scheduled insulin therapy with subsequent intensification of therapy, based upon patients' response to treatment. Sliding scales alone should be discouraged secondary to the availability of more effective treatment alternatives. Availability of prospective, randomized trials that shed light on the impact of tight or improved glucose control on morbidity and mortality in the non-intensive care unit setting should be undertaken. The presence of hyperglycemia in diabetic and non-diabetic patients needs to be addressed with the implementation of appropriate treatment regimens that have been shown to avoid hyperglycemia.

# References

1. Joslin EP. *A Diabetic Manual for the Mutual Use of Doctor and Patient.* Philadelphia, Lea & Febiger, 1934;108.

2. Marks V. Blood glucose: its measurement and clinical importance. *Clin Chim Acta* 1996;251:3-17.

3. Skyler JS, Skyler DL, Seigler DE, O'Sullivan MJ. Algorithms for adjustment of insulin dosage by patients who monitor blood glucose. *Diabetes Care* 1981;4:311-318.

4. Skyler JS. Intensive insulin therapy: a personal and historical perspective. *Diabetes Educ* 1989;15:33-39.

5. Pernick NL, Rodbard D. Personal computer programs to assist with self-monitoring of blood glucose and self-adjustment of insulin dosage. *Diabetes Care* 1986;9:61-69.

6. Umpierrez GE, Palacio A, Smiley D. Sliding scale insulin use: Myth or insanity? The *Am J Med* 2007;120:563-567.

7. Browning LA, Dumo P. Sliding-scale insulin: an antiquated approach to glycemic control in hospitalized patients. *Am J Health-Syst Pharm* 2004;61:1611-1614.

8. Levetan CS, Magee MF. Hospital management of diabetes. *Endocrinol Metab Clin North Am* 2000;29:745-770.

9. Clement S, Braithwaite SS, Magee MF, et al. Management of diabetes and hyperglycemia in hospitals. *Diabetes Care* 2004;27:553-597.

10. UK Prospective Diabetes Study Group. Intensive blood-glucose control with sulfonylureas or insulin compared with conventional treatment. *Lancet* 1998;352:837-53.

11. Umpierrez GE, Isaac SD, Bazargan N, et al. Hyperglycemia: and independent marker of in-hospital mortality in patients with undiagnosed diabetes. *J Clin Endocrinol Metab* 2002;87:978-982.

12. Pomposelli JJ, Baxter JK, Babineau TJ, et al. Early postoperative predicts nosocomial infection rate in diabetic patients. *J Parenter Enteral Nutr* 1998;22:77-81.

13. ACE Position Statement on Inpatient Diabetes and Metabolic Control. *Endocr Pract* 2004;10:78-82.

14. Queale WS, Seidler AJ, Brancati FL. Glycemic control and sliding scale insulin use in medical in patients with diabetes mellitus. *Arch Intern Med* 1997;157:545-552.

15. Golightly LK, Jones MA, Hamamura DH, et al. Management of diabetes mellitus in hospitalized patients: Efficiency and effectiveness of sliding-scale insulin therapy. *Pharmacotherapy* 2006;26:1421–1432.

16. Umpierrez GE, Palacio A, Smiley D. Randomized study of basal-bolus insulin therapy in the inpatient management of patients with type 2 diabetes (RABBIT 2 Trial). *Diabetes Care* 2007;30:2181-2185.

17. Matheny ME, Shubina M, Kimmel ZM, et al. Treatment intensification and blood glucose control among hospitalized diabetic patients. *J Gen Intern Med* 2007;23:184-189.

18. Cefalu WT. Pharmacotherapy for the Treatment of Patients with Type 2 Diabetes Mellitus: Rationale and Specific Agents. *Clin Pharmacol Therap* 2007;81:636-649.

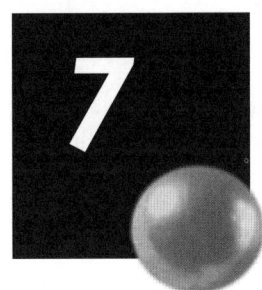

# 7

# Glycemic Control in the ICU: How Low Should We Go?

*Debra J. Skaar*

## Background and Introduction

Emerging evidence strongly associates even modest hyperglycemia in critically ill patients with poorer outcomes.[1,2] As recent as the 1990s, most clinicians treated stress hyperglycemia in hospitalized patients only when blood glucose measurements exceeded 180-200 mg/dL. The landmark study by Van den Berghe published in 2001 challenged this practice by demonstrating that intensive insulin therapy to maintain blood glucose between 80-110 mg/dL improved outcomes in critically ill patients.[3]

This single-center Belgium study (commonly referred to as the Leuven I study) in critically ill, mechanically ventilated, surgical intensive care unit (ICU) patients, 2/3 cardiac, compared conventional management of hyperglycemia (blood glucose maintained between 180-200 mg/dL) to an intensive treatment arm (blood glucose maintained between 80-110 mg/dL) both with a continuous insulin infusion. Both ICU and hospital survival was significantly improved with intensive insulin treatment (IIT) versus the conventional insulin treatment (CIT), (ICU survival 4.6% vs. 8%, p=0.005; Hospital survival 16.8% vs. 26.3%, p=0.01) (Fig. 7.1) For patients requiring more than 5 days of ICU care, intensive glycemic control improved mortality from 20.2% to 10.6% (p=0.07). In addition, IIT was also associated with a significant reduction in a host of secondary outcomes: ICU length of stay, days of mechanical ventilation, acute renal failure requiring dialysis, septicemia, hyperbilirubinemia, and critical-illness polyneuropathy. Other investigators noted that hospitalized patients with new hyperglycemia were more likely to be admitted to the ICU, have a longer length of stay, and less likely to be discharged home than either known diabetics or normoglycemic patients. Another study demonstrated increased mortality at each APACHE II range with higher blood glucose values in a mixed medical/surgical ICU. Blood glucose values of 80-139 mg/dL were associated with the lowest mortality, 9.6-15.1%, whereas patients with blood glucose measurements exceeding 300 mg/dL had a mortality of 42.5%.[3]

In a separate analysis of her original study, Van den Berghe determined that glycemic control, not insulin dose, was associated with mortality benefit. For groups comparable at baseline, patients who had blood glucose levels less than 110 mg/dL, mortality was <15%; whereas patients with blood glucose levels ranging between 110-150 mg had 25% mortality; and in patients whose blood glucose levels were over 150 mg, mortality approached 40%.[4] These findings were corroborated by Finney who reported that glycemic control (blood glucose <145 mg/dL) was the factor associated with lower mortality, not insulin dosage.[5]

The importance of glycemic control suddenly became a hot and controversial topic among ICU clinicians. Remarkable improvements in morbidity and mortality possible with tight glycemic control could be offered to many critically ill patients, not a treatment limited to patients with sepsis or MI. Unfortunately, the Leuven study has been criticized for a number of limitations. The single-center study was conducted in a surgical ICU primarily in patients who had undergone cardiac surgery who had a higher than usual mortality (5.1%) in the control group. Patients in the study had received more glucose calories (200-300 gm/d) and parenteral nutrition than is recommended in the USA. The IIT may have caused its beneficial effects by decreasing the adverse effect of this high glucose load. The study was not blinded so the IIT group could have received better care than the CIT group. Insulin dosage adjustments were done by a separate team of physicians/nurses, a scenario not consistent with clinical practice where a severe nursing shortage can limit the time nurses have to monitor and adjust insulin infusions to keep blood glucose within a tight range. Potential benefits must be weighed against questions yet unanswered.

## How Have Critical Care Pharmacists Changed Their Practice?

A survey of critical care pharmacists who were members of the American College of Clinical Pharmacy Practice and Research Network (crit-PRN) was emailed in August 2003 to assess how the Leuven study had affected their ICU's glycemic goals. The initial questionnaire

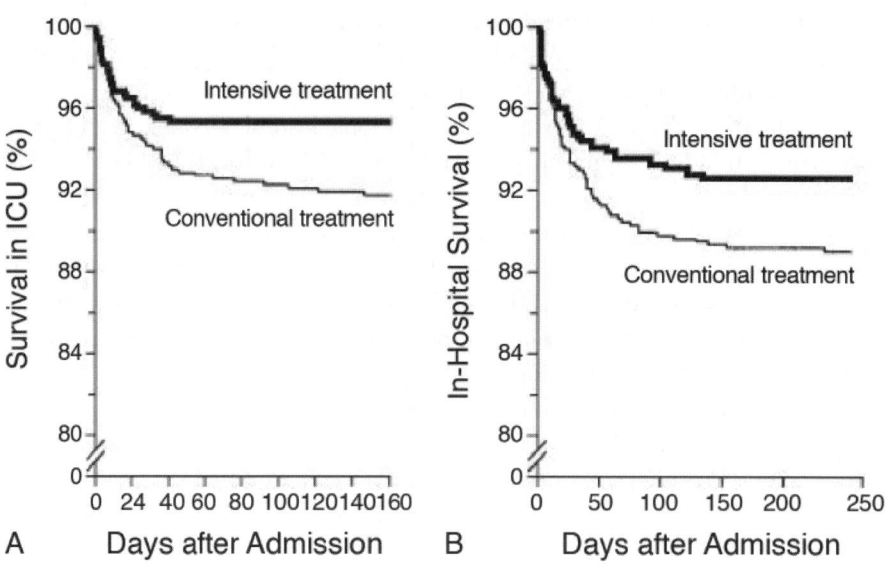

**Figure 7.1.** Kaplan–Meier curves showing cumulative survival of patients who received intensive insulin treatment or conventional treatment in the intensive care unit (ICU) from Leuven I. Patients discharged alive from the ICU (Panel A) and from the hospital (Panel B) were considered to have survived. In both cases, the differences between the treatment groups were significant (survival in ICU, nominal p=0.005 and adjusted p<0.04; in-hospital survival, nominal p=0.01). P values were determined with the use of the Mantel–Cox log-rank test.

contained only six questions; electronic reminders were sent out twice within a month to maximize response rate. All except one of the 50 critical care pharmacists who responded to the survey were familiar with the Leuven study and had altered their management of hyperglycemia based on the study's results. In 2003, over 30% had selected 80-110 mg/dL as their ICU's target range. The rest implemented tighter ranges of glycemic control but with lower acceptable targets ranging from 51 mg/dL to greater than 120 mg/dL and the upper acceptable target varying from 120 mg/dL to greater than 150 mg/dL. Nursing staffing and education was voiced as the most significant barrier to implementing an intensive insulin protocol, followed by challenges in interpretation and implementation of the protocol, physician acceptance, and fear of hypoglycemia, respectively.

In April 2005, a second email survey was sent to the "early adopters" to assess if they had altered their glycemic goals and/or protocols based on clinical practice and/or emerging scientific evidence. Nearly half of intensive care units surveyed had not changed their intensive insulin protocols in any way since implementation in 2003. Based on their hospital's experience and outcome data demonstrating positive results without increasing concerns of hypoglycemia, a third of critical care pharmacists responding had tightened up their target glycemic range most commonly to an upper acceptable target ≤ 120 mg/dL. Some protocols required refinements with hospital system changes to improve ease of interpretation and implementation. Only one pharmacist's ICU had altered their target range to a less intense glycemic control.

## Intensive Insulin in the Medical ICU

In early 2006, the long-awaited medical ICU study (Leuven II) found somewhat different reductions in morbidity and no mortality benefit among a medical ICU patient population. The study methods were similar to that of Leuven I except insulin dosage adjustments based on blood glucose levels were made by bedside nurses in the ICU, not research nurses and physicians. Reduced morbidity in the IIT group compared to CIT patients included newly acquired kidney injury, earlier weaning from mechanical ventilation, and a reduced ICU and hospital length of stay. There was no statistically significant benefit from tight glycemic control on bacteremia, prolonged use of antibiotics, or TISS-28 scores. Mortality was not reduced by IIT compared to CIT (37.3% vs. 40%; p=0.33) in the medical ICU unless the ICU length of stay was greater than or equal to 3 days (43% vs. 52%; p=0.009), a factor that cannot be reliably predicted at admission (Fig. 7.2).

Hypoglycemia (blood glucose levels ≤ 40 mg/dL) occurred more frequently in the IIT group than the CIT. Despite the use of similar insulin titration guidelines, an episode of hypoglycemia occurred more frequently in the medical ICU study than the surgical study.[6] Patients in the medical ICU study were more critically ill, as evidenced by the high mortality rate, 38.6%. Increasing severity of illness increases the likelihood of severe hypoglycemia, and severe hypoglycemia has been shown to double the risk of death.[7]

## Conflicting Results and Controversies

Several other groups attempted to replicate the Leuven results with conflicting results. A multicenter German study, VISEP (Efficacy of Volume Substitution and Insulin Therapy in Severe Sepsis), was designed to evaluate 600 critically ill medical or surgical patients with severe sepsis who were randomized to intensive or conventional insulin therapy. Recruitment was stopped early due to safety reasons, no difference in mortality, and more frequent hypoglycemia.[8] The IIT group had a higher rate of severe hypoglycemia (glucose level $\leq$ 40 mg/dL) than the CIT group (17% vs. 4.1%; p<0.001), and their rate of serious adverse events was also higher (10.9% vs. 5.2%; p=0.01).[9] The Glucontrol study, designed to randomize 3,500 medical and surgical ICU patients in Europe, to tight or modest blood glucose control was also suspended after the first interim analysis due to increased mortality and marked hypoglycemia in the IIT group (8.6%).[10] Although target glycemic goals in these studies were not attained, patients had a higher risk for hypoglycemia and adverse outcomes. Neither study was powered for statistical significance since they were stopped before completion. Figure 7.3 shows the incidence of severe hypoglycemia reported in seven studies.[11]

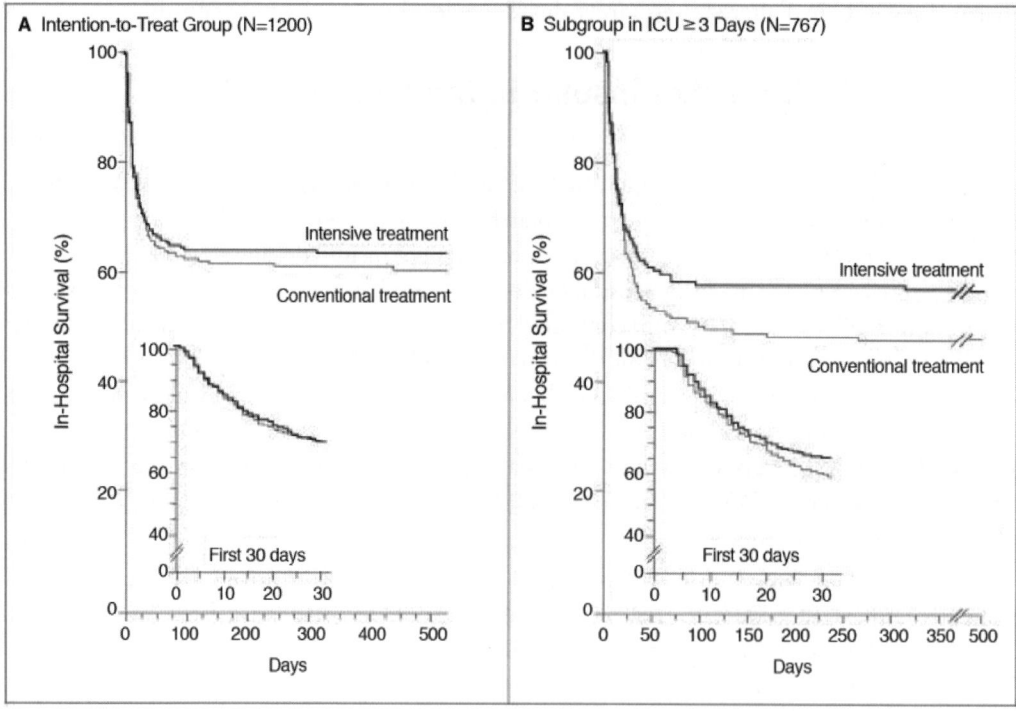

**Figure 7.2.** Kaplan–Meier curves for in-hospital survival from Leuven II (MICU). The effect of intensive insulin treatment on the time from admission to the intensive care unit (ICU) until death is shown for the intention-to-treat group (Panel A) and the subgroup of patients staying in the ICU for 3 or more days (Panel B). Patients discharged alive from the hospital were considered survivors. P values calculated by the log-rank test were 0.40 for the intention-to-treat group and 0.02 for the subgroup staying in the ICU for three or more days. P values calculated by proportional-hazards regression analysis were 0.30 and 0.02, respectively.

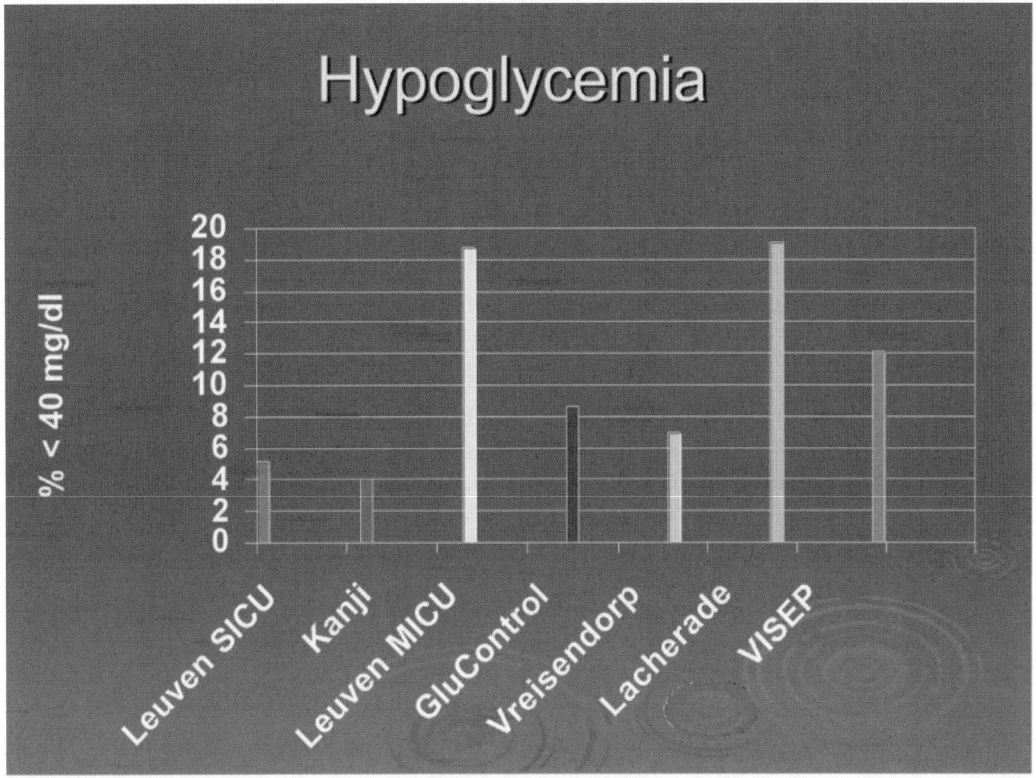

**Figure 7.3.** Hypoglycemia rates from selected studies of tight glycemic control.

Additional studies have identified risk factors for hypoglycemia and poor outcomes. Vreisendorp and colleagues found preexisting diabetes mellitus, dialysis, sepsis, and use of insulin to predispose critically ill patients to hypoglycemia. Failure to adjust insulin dose when reducing nutrition was also a risk factor for hypoglycemia.[12] A database of over 5,000 patients identified 102 patients with an episode of severe hypoglycemia. Multivariate logistic regression analysis identified diabetes, septic shock, inotropic support, renal insufficiency, mechanical ventilation, severity of illness, and treatment with tight glycemic control as independent risk factors for hypoglycemia. Mortality was higher in the patients with hypoglycemia than the control group (55.9% vs. 39.5%, p=0.0057). A sensitivity analysis suggested that the mortality benefit of tight glycemic control outweighed the mortality attributed to severe hypoglycemia.[7]

Why are clinicians so concerned about transient hypoglycemia? The brain requires a constant source of glucose for energy since it cannot store or synthesize glucose. Neuroglycopenia has been shown to be harmful. Imaging studies have demonstrated anatomical alterations in patients with sustained hypoglycemia. No long-term studies have been done to evaluate the potential neurocognitive damage caused by minutes or hours of severe hypoglycemia.[11]

A French group recently reported increased (22.2% vs. 50%; p=0.006) ICU mortality when glycemic control was not achieved and even higher mortality when glycemic control is lost after initial control in a medical ICU (23.3% vs. 56.2%; p=0.002). The odds ratio for ICU death was greater than 3 in patients whose blood glucose was not controlled and almost 6 in the group who lost glycemic control after initial hyperglycemic correction.[13]

## Has Clinical Practice Changed with Leuven II and New Scientific Data?

Critical care pharmacists were asked in November 2007 if their target glycemic goals had changed in response to findings from the medical ICU study (Leuven II) and other tight glycemic control studies that were stopped prematurely at interim analysis (e.g., VISEP, Glucontrol). Pharmacists were requested to share their current target range and reasons for any changes within the past 18 months. Survey results from approximately 50 pharmacists suggested that practice had not changed significantly since the results of Leuven II were published in 2006 (Fig. 7.4). Only two pharmacists indicated that their target range had increased slightly (to 90-145 mg/dL) as of late 2007. Protocol revision was common to facilitate systems changes, and reported rates of

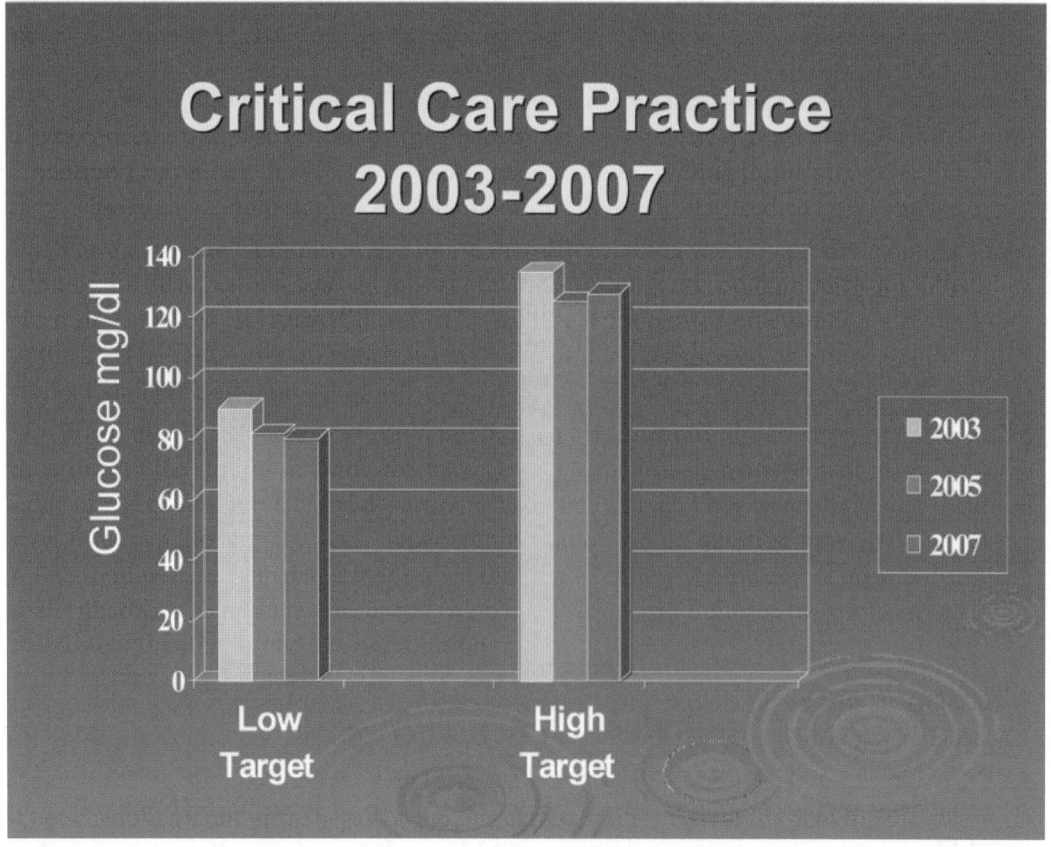

**Figure 7.4.** Changes in target glycemic goals in critical care practice from 2003-2007.

hypoglycemia were low (<1%) with intensive insulin protocols. Most pharmacists stated that their ICU teams were waiting for the results of the NICE-SUGAR study before implementing changes in their glycemic goals.

## NICE-SUGAR

The Normoglycemia in Intensive Care Evaluation and Survival Using Glucose Algorithm Regulation Study (NICE-SUGAR Study) is a multicenter (over 35 ICUs from Australia, New Zealand, Canada, and USA), open-label, randomized controlled trial of blood glucose management with IIT to maintain blood glucose between 4.5-6.0 mmol/L (81-108 mg/dL) versus a less intensive insulin regimen targeting blood glucose level between 8-10 mmol/L (144-180 mg/dL). The study's primary outcome is 90-day all-cause mortality with secondary outcomes including ICU and hospital mortality, length of ICU and hospital stay, need for organ support (inotropes, dialysis and positive pressure ventilation), blood stream infections, incidence and severity of hypoglycemia, and long-term functional status for a subgroup of patients with traumatic brain injury. Enrollment for the first 5300 patients is complete. The Canadian (SUGAR) started later and continues to enroll toward a goal of 6,100 total patients.[14]

## Conclusion

*Tighter* glycemic control has been shown to reduce morbidity and mortality in critically ill patients. *How low should we go* to maximize positive outcomes and minimize the risk of severe hypoglycemia remains controversial. The 2008 Sepsis Campaign Guidelines recommend IV insulin therapy in patients with severe sepsis to reduce hyperglycemia and suggests target glucose levels <150 mg/dL using a validated protocol for insulin dose adjustments. In addition, this consensus conference recommends blood glucose monitoring every 1-2 hours until glucose values and insulin infusion rates are stable and then every 4 hours. Low glucose levels obtained with point-of-care testing on capillary blood may overestimate arterial blood or plasma glucose levels and must be interpreted with caution.[15] With several studies linking severe hypoglycemia to poor outcomes and death, identifying and quickly managing low glucose levels must be included in every insulin protocol. Most intensive care clinicians are continuing with the protocols they have successfully implemented in their ICUs and using intensive insulin therapy for tight glycemic control (blood glucose target range 80-110 mg/dL) until the results of the NICE-SUGAR study are published.

## References

1. Umpierrez GE, Isaacs SD, Bazargan N, et al. Hyperglycemia: an independent marker of in-hospital mortality in patients with undiagnosed diabetes. *J Clin Endocrinol Metab* 2002:87;978-982.
2. Krinsley JS. Association between hyperglycemia and increased hospital mortality in a heterogeneous population of critically ill patients. *Mayo Clin Proceed* 2003;78:1471-1478.
3. Van den Berghe G, Wouters P, Weekers F, et al. Intensive insulin therapy in critically ill patients. *N Engl J Med* 2001;345:1359-1367.

4. Van den Berghe G, Wouters PJ, Bouillon R, et al. Outcome benefit of intensive insulin therapy in the critically ill: insulin dose versus glycemic control. *Crit Care Med* 2003;31:359-366.

5. Finney SJ, Zekveld C, Elia A, et al. Glucose control and mortality in critically ill patients. *JAMA* 2003;290:2041-2047.

6. Van den Berghe G, Willmer, A, Hermans G, et al. Intensive insulin therapy in the medical ICU. *N Engl J Med* 2006;354:449-461.

7. Krinsley J, Grover A. Severe hypoglycemia in critically ill patients: risk factors and outcomes. *Crit Care Med* 2007;35:2262-2267.

8. Brunkhorst FM, Kuhnt E, Engel C, et al. Intensive insulin therapy in patients with severe sepsis and septic shock ins associated with an increased rate of hypoglycemia-results from a randomized multicenter study (VISEP). *Infection* 2005;33(Suppl 1);19.

9. Brunkhorst FM, Engel C, Bloos F, et al. Intensive insulin therapy and pentastarch resuscitation in severe sepsis. *N Engl J Med* 2008;358;2:125-139.

10. Preiser JC. Intensive glycemic control in med-surg patients (European Glucontrol trial). Paper presented at: Society of Critical Care Medicine 36th Critical Care Congress; February 17-21, 2007;Orlando, FL.

11. Nasraway SA. Sitting on the horns of a dilemma: avoiding severe hypoglycemia while practicing tight glycemic control. *Crit Care Med* 2007;35(10):2435-2437.

12. Vreisendorp TM, DeVries JH, van Santen, et al. Predisposing factors for hypoglycemia in the intensive care unit. *Crit Care Med* 2006;34:96-101.

13. Lacherade JC, Jabre P, Bastuji-Garin S, et al. *Intl Care Med* 2007;33:814-821.

14. The George Institute, Normoglycaemia in Intensive Care Evaluation and Survival Using Glucose Algorithm Study - NICE-SUGAR. Available at: http://www.thegeorgeinstitute. org/research/critical-care-&-trauma/research/normoglycaemia-in-intensive-care-evaluation---nice.cfm. Accessed May 27, 2008.

15. Dellinger RP, Levy MM, Carlet JM, et al. Surviving sepsis campaign: international guidelines for management of severe sepsis and septic shock: 2008. *Intl Care Med* 2008;34:17-60.

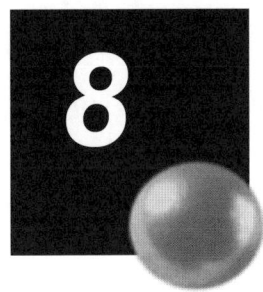

# ASAP: Aspirin-Use Screen for Acute Myocardial Infarction Patients

*Hoytin T. Lee Ghin*

## Introduction

Each year more than 1 million Americans have a heart attack, approximately 800 thousand new and 500 thousand recurrent,[1,3] and approximately a third of these patients do not survive.[1-3] The Institute for Healthcare Improvement, a not-for-profit organization, which focuses on improving worldwide healthcare, launched the 100,000 lives campaign – a national initiative, with a goal of saving 100,000 lives among patients in hospitals through improvements in the safety and effectiveness of health care. One of the key components of this campaign is "fast and effective acute myocardial infarction (AMI) care." The 100,000 lives campaign was so successful it is now the 5 million lives campaign. Fast and effective AMI care has also been identified as an important area for improvement by both The Joint Commission and the Centers for Medicare and Medicaid Services.[3]

Both the American College of Cardiology (ACC) and the American Heart Association (AHA) consider the items listed in Table 8.1 to be key components of optimal AMI care.[2,4,5]

### Table 8.1. ACC/AHA Key Components of Optimal AMI Care [2,4,5]

- Early administration of aspirin (within 24 hours)
- Aspirin at discharge
- Early administration of beta-blocker
- Beta-blocker at discharge
- ACE-inhibitor or ARB at discharge for patients with systolic dysfunction
- Timely initiation of reperfusion (thrombolysis or percutaneous intervention)
- Smoking cessation counseling

The top two components involve aspirin. The first item, early administration of aspirin is the subject of this pearl.

## Benefits of Aspirin

The benefits of aspirin administration within the first 24 hours were demonstrated in the ISIS-2 trial. In the ISIS-2 trial, aspirin administration, within 24 hours, prevented 10 nonfatal re-infarctions and 3 nonfatal strokes per 1,000 patients treated. The effects of aspirin were uniform in both early and late presenters of AMI, and the benefit of initial aspirin therapy was sustained long-term. Because of these benefits, the administration of aspirin within the first 24 hours is considered a Class IA recommendation by both the ACC and AHA.[4,5]

## National Quality or Core Measures

Although this process is both simple and effective, not 100% of eligible patients receive aspirin within the first 24 hours. The nationwide average for compliance on this measure is 93%.[7]

There is currently a nationwide push for standardization of healthcare administration; and as a result, the national quality measures were formed. Hospitals will be graded on and compared with other institutions on these quality measures, analogous to The Joint Commission Accreditation status. Most states will make hospitals' record cards public information. As a result, hospitals ensure adherence to these measures through their Performance Improvement (PI) Department.

By collaborating with the PI department, not only can pharmacists assist in ensuring compliance with these quality measures, they can directly impact patient care.

### Table 8.2. AMI-Aspirin Screen Basic Chart Review

**Who should get:**

- Any patient suspected of ACS, (+) EKG changes, (+) troponins.

**Who should not get:**

- Documented serious allergic reaction

- Recent severe GI bleeding or suspected ICH

# Screening Process

Depending on the institution, the screening process may only take a few minutes. The process at our institution is as follows:

1. A patient list is generated by the PI department.
2. Review patient chart.
3. Contact the physician, if necessary, to initiate therapy.

The most time consuming part of this process is reading the patient's chart, looking for exclusion criteria. Most, if not all, physicians would be responsive to initiating aspirin therapy. After contacting the physician, if he/she does not believe aspirin would be beneficial for the patient at this time, all the physician has to do is document their reason in their progress note to be in compliance with this national quality measure.

A basic chart review guide that lists who should and should not get aspirin is provided in Table 8.2. Ensuring that patients get aspirin, if needed, is a simple intervention with potentially significant impact on patient care.

# Conclusion

Pharmacists may tend to think of collaborative practice as a collaboration with physicians only; however, it can be applied in broader terms to a true health-care team approach to improve patient care. The aforementioned process is a simple and easy approach to ensure appropriate aspirin administration. A similar process can be applied to any national quality measure,[8] e.g., appropriate use of antibiotics for pneumonia or ACE inhibitors or ARBs in patients with LV dysfunction. The Performance Improvement Department is one resource where pharmacists can get involved in improving patient care, both directly and indirectly.

# References

1. Rosamond W, Flegal K, Friday G, et al. Heart disease and stroke statistics—2007 update: a report from the American Heart Association Statistics Committee and Stroke Statistics Subcommittee. *Circulation* 2007;115(5):e69-e171.
2. Berwick DM, Calkins DR, McCannon CJ, et al. The 100,000 lives campaign: setting a goal and a deadline for improving health care quality. *JAMA* 2006;295:324-327.
3. Institute for Healthcare Improvement. When Every minute Counts: Improving Heart Attack Care. Available at: http://www.ihi.org/IHI/Topics/Reliability/ReliabilityGeneral/ImprovementStories/WhenEveryMinuteCountsImprovingHeartAttackCare.html. Accessed October 31, 2007.
4. Antman EM, Anbe DT, Armstrong PW, et al. ACC/AHA guidelines for the management of patients with ST-elevation myocardial infarction-executive summary. A report of the American College of Cardiology/American Heart Association Task Force on Practice Guidelines (Writing Committee to revise the 1999 guidelines for the management of patients with acute myocardial infarction). *J Am Coll Cardiol* 2004;44(3):671-719.

5. Anderson JL, Adams CD, Antman EM, et al. ACC/AHA 2007 guidelines for the management of patients with unstable angina/non-ST-Elevation myocardial infarction: a report of the American College of Cardiology/American Heart Association Task Force on Practice Guidelines (Writing Committee to Revise the 2002 Guidelines for the Management of Patients With Unstable Angina/Non-ST-Elevation Myocardial Infarction) developed in collaboration with the American College of Emergency Physicians, the Society for Cardiovascular Angiography and Interventions, and the Society of Thoracic Surgeons endorsed by the American Association of Cardiovascular and Pulmonary Rehabilitation and the Society for Academic Emergency Medicine. *J Am Coll Cordiol* 2007;50(7):e1-e157.

6. United States Department of Health & Human Services. Hospital Compare Webpage. Available from: http://www.hospitalcompare.hhs.gov. Accessed October 31, 2007.

7. Baigent C, Collins R, Appleby P, et al. ISIS-2:10 year survival among patients with suspected acute myocardial infarction in randomised comparison of intravenous streptokinase, oral aspirin, both, or neither. *Br Med J* 1998;316(7141):1337-43.

8. United States Department of Health & Human Services. Hospital Process of Care Measure Set Webpage. Available from: http://www.hospitalcompare.hhs.gov/Hospital/Static/Data-Professionals.asp?dest=NAV|Home|DataDetails|ProfessionalInfo#measureset. Accessed on October 31, 2007.

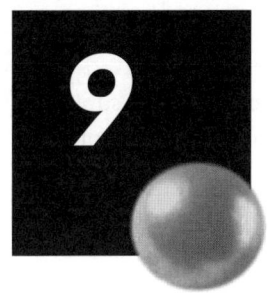

# Soy, You Want to Be a Girlie Man? Effect of Soy Supplementation on Testosterone in Healthy Males

*Susan Goodin*

## Background and Introduction

Soy is a dietary staple consumed in Asia for more than 5,000 years. Soy products, which are high in protein, are consumed in numerous forms including soybeans, soy milk, miso, tofu, and soy sauce, to name a few. The popularity of soy products in the United States has increased over the years as consumers have pursued healthier lifestyles. The early interest in soy consumption was further motivated by the US Food and Drug Administration (FDA) approved labeling for foods containing soy protein as protective against coronary heart disease.[1] Although generally viewed as healthy, consumption has been associated with a number of controversial and undefined health outcomes. The presence of isoflavones, and their estrogenic activity, in soy protein preparations led to the investigation of soy effects on decreasing the risk of prostate cancer due to their ability to decrease testosterone.

## Soy and Health Outcomes

Early interest in the health effects of soy was based on its potential role in improving risk factors for cardiovascular disease. A meta-analysis of the effects of soy protein intake on serum lipids published in 1995 reported a significant reduction on total cholesterol, LDL cholesterol, and triglycerides and a non-significant increase in HDL cholesterol.[2] This and other studies led to the FDA health claim for labeling of foods in 1999 that both total and LDL cholesterol can be lowered by consuming 25 grams per day of soy protein.[1] The FDA requires for the claim that a serving contain at least 6.25 g of soy protein, 25% of the necessary daily amount, with the expectation that foods containing soy protein would be eaten at least four times a day. Importantly, the FDA health claim stated that the evidence did not support a significant role for soy isoflavones in lowering cholesterol. A year later, the American Heart Association recommended that patients with elevated cholesterol include soy protein foods in their diet.[3] Since then, many well-controlled studies have substantially added to our understanding of the role of soy protein and soy-derived isoflavones in cardiovascular disease. A more recent meta-analysis in which investigators reported a relatively small effect of soy protein on cholesterol actually supported the FDAs claim regarding the lack of a significant effect of isoflavones in lowering cholesterol and preventing cardiovascular disease. [4]

Despite the numerous studies of soy in preventing several diseases, more recently a government report has concluded that there is limited evidence supporting the health benefits of soy in reducing the risk of heart disease, as well as several other diseases.[5] An analysis funded by the Agency for Healthcare Research and Quality (AHRQ) evaluated 178 prospective studies of soy foods, soymilk, and soy supplements, including extracts of isoflavones. The review included evaluation of soy's effect on bone health, kidney disease, endocrine function, reproductive health, neurocognitive function, glucose metabolism, heart disease, and cancer. While the review team concluded that soy consumption seemed to offer only small benefits in reducing the risk of heart disease and hot flashes during menopause, the results were inconclusive for several diseases including cancer.

## Soy Effects on Testosterone

Soy has been suggested as an agent for the prevention of cancer since higher testosterone levels are considered a potential risk factor for prostate cancer by the National Cancer Institute. The benefit of soy for cancer prevention may be from a decrease in testosterone. Investigation into the hormonal effects from soy has been proposed because of the presence of isoflavones. Isoflavones found in soy include genistein and daidzein and are believed to have estrogen-like effects; therefore, they are often referred to as phytoestrogens. Genistein and daidzein are structurally similar to endogenous estrogen (Fig. 9.1) and are ligands to estrogen receptors alpha and beta, with a weaker affinity than endogenous estrogen, resulting in estrogenic and anti-estrogenic effects. The resulting hormonal effects for binding to the estrogen receptor are dependent on the individual's amount of circulating endogenous estrogens and the type and number of receptors in the target tissues.

All soy products do not contain the same amount of isoflavones, and depending on how they are extracted, may contain no isoflavones.[6] The amount of isoflavones present in a soy product may determine the hormonal effects when consumed. Additionally, beyond the amount of

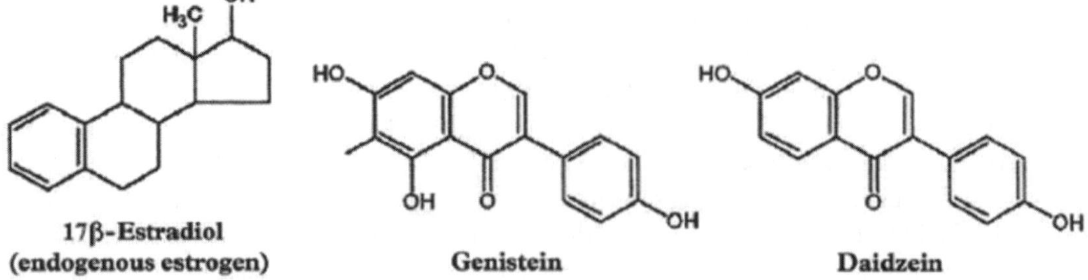

**Figure 9.1.** Chemical structures of the phytoestrogens genestein, daidzein, and endogenous estrogen, 17 β–estradiol.

isoflavone present, the interaction of the isoflavone at the estrogen receptor varies with different formulations of soy, resulting in variable effects on the production of estrogen.[7] Each of these factors effect the hormonal action of soy protein products. Beyond the structural relationship, other support for the hormonal effects of soy include their inhibition of steroid biosynthetic enzymes, and numerous animal studies reporting reduced serum androgens fed isoflavones at various concentrations in numerous formulations.[8-10]

While there is increased interest in the hormonal effects of soy, few studies have assessed the hormonal effects of soy supplementation in healthy men. Clinically, to evaluate the estrogen effects of soy in men, assessment of testosterone in men has been the primary endpoint because the consumption of estrogen should result in a reduction in testosterone.

To assess the effects of dietary intake without additional supplementation, Nagata et. al.[11] performed a cross-sectional analysis of the relationship between soy product intake and reproductive hormones. Their dietary questionnaire assessment of 69 Japanese men, mean age of 60.5 years, reported an inverse correlation between soyfood consumption and serum estradiol after controlling for age, body mass index, smoking status, and ethanol intake. A borderline significant association between soyfood consumption and serum estrone, total testosterone, and free testosterone was also reported. Average isoflavone intake was estimated to be 22 mg/d, although the authors reported that diet records estimated soy intake to be 40% higher.

Prospective dietary intervention studies have included the evaluation of the effects of tofu,[12] soymilk,[13,14] soy extract,[15] soy protein isolates,[16,17] soya flour scones,[18] and soy protein powder[19] on testosterone in healthy men. The initial trial to evaluate a dietary supplement was a randomized crossover study of 42 men, with a mean age of 45.7 years, that assessed the effects of 4 weeks of 150 g of lean meat or 290 g of tofu containing approximately 70 mg of isoflavones.[12] Although a slight reduction in androgen activity was reported, there was not a statistically significant reduction in testosterone.

The effect of soymilk supplementation has been evaluated in two separate trials.[13,14] In a parallel-arm study of 34 men, with a mean age of 32.4 years, of which half of the subjects consumed an average of 343 mL of soymilk containing approximately 48 mg of isoflavones for 8 weeks, there were no differences in testosterone levels between the groups.[13] In a cross-sectional analysis of 696 men with varying intakes of soymilk, soy milk intake was measured using a validated semi-quantitative food frequency questionnaire.[14] Again there was no association of soy intake with decreased testosterone. The results of soymilk supplementation are consistent with those reported with the use of a tablet containing 40 mg/day for 8 weeks.[15] Finally, the largest study evaluating the effects of soy on testosterone levels was a placebo-controlled trial of soy protein isolate, containing 118 mg of isoflavone, or casein placebo for 12 weeks. In the 55 men, median age of 61 years (range, 50-75 years), there was no effect on testosterone levels.[16]

Three trials have reported a statistically significant decrease in testosterone with soy supplementation.[17-19] In a randomized, cross-over design, 30 men, mean age 27.9 years, consumed milk protein isolate (MPI), low-isoflavone soy protein isolate, and high-isoflavone soy protein isolate for 8 weeks. Statistically significant decreases in testosterone by the low-isoflavone soy protein isolate occurred relative to the MPI and high-isoflavone soy protein isolate at 29 days but not at 57 days.[17] Similarly, in a placebo-controlled cross-over trial of 20 healthy males, mean age of 35.6 years, three soya scones a day, containing 120 mg/day of isoflavones, for 6 weeks was associated with a statistically significant decrease in testosterone (p=0.03).[18] Finally, a recent study in 12 healthy males, mean age of 32.25 years, receiving soy protein powder containing an unknown amount of isoflavones for 4 weeks resulted in a statistically significant (p=0.021) decrease in testosterone.[19]

Eight studies with a total of 212 participants have reported testosterone levels in healthy males before and after soy consumption.[12-19] Five of these trials found a statistically non-significant decrease in testosterone levels, whereas three studies reported a statistically significant decrease in testosterone. Among all the trials, there was no correlation with the amount of isoflavone content and lowering of testosterone. Possible explanations for a lack of demonstrated testosterone change in studies could be the heterogeneity in the soy products that were used in each of the studies. Consequently, it may not be the phytoestrogen content

## Table 9.1. Studies Evaluating the Effect of Soy Protein on Testosterone in Healthy Males

| Soy Formulation | Subjects | Isoflavone Content (mg/day) | Duration (weeks) | Mean age of subjects (years) | Statistically Significant Decrease in Testosterone? |
|---|---|---|---|---|---|
| Tofu[12] | 42 | 70 | 4 | 45.7 | No |
| Soymilk[13] | 34 | 48 | 8 | 32.4 | No |
| Soy extract tablet[15] | 14 | 40 | 8 | NR Range: 18-35 | No |
| Soy protein isolate[16] | 55 | 118 | 13.5 | 61 | No |
| High-soy isoflavone protein isolate[17] | 35 | $61.6 \pm 7.35$ | 8 | 27.9 | No |
| Low-soy isoflavone protein isolate[17] | 35 | $1.64 \pm 0.19$ | 8 | 27.9 | Yes* – 10% |
| Soya flour scones[18] | 20 | 120 | 6 | 35.6 | Yes – 6% |
| Soy protein powder[19] | 12 | NR | 4 | 32.25 | Yes – 19% |

*At day 29, but not at end of study.
NR: Not reported.

but possibly the selectivity for the estrogen receptor type that is important in the effects on testosterone. Additionally, due to the daily variation in testosterone levels, if not adequately controlled, outcomes are greatly affected. Future studies must rigorously control for soy use and the effects of soy on testosterone during and after stopping supplementation.

## Consequences of Low Testosterone

The relationship between endogenous testosterone and health in men is controversial. Early concerns were that decreased testosterone may result in a decline in sperm quality at high doses or when consumed for long periods.[15,20] While supplementation with a tablet of 40 mg/day of soy isoflavones for 8 weeks had no effects on testicular or ejaculate volume or sperm concentration, count, or motility, the investigators noted that effects from exposure during development or consumption of higher doses for a longer period are unknown and not answered by their study.[15] Conversely, a recent meta-analysis noted that testosterone supplementation in patients with low testosterone is associated with only a small improvement in erectile function so the effect of soy on lowering testosterone may play little role in sexual function.[21]

Other possible consequences of reduced testosterone levels include osteoporosis, adverse cardiovascular risk factors, systolic and diastolic hypertension, obesity, insulin resistance, and increased fibrinogen levels.[22] In fact, a recent case-controlled study in more than 11,000 British men, ages 40-79 with no cardiovascular risk factors, revealed that low testosterone may be a predictive marker for cardiovascular disease.[23] The patients in the upper 25 percent of testosterone concentrations had a 41% lower risk of death from heart attack, stroke, and other cardiovascular conditions. Similarly, another study of approximately 800 men reported that patients with the lowest testosterone levels were 40 percent more likely to die.[24] Regardless of the lack of consistent data regarding the role of soy in decreasing testosterone, all men should be questioned about soy supplementation, and testosterone levels should be assessed in men reporting a positive history of use.

While a higher testosterone level is considered a potential risk factor for prostate cancer, it is unclear that a decrease in testosterone translates to a decrease in prostate cancer risk. In African American men, mean age 20.6 years, testosterone levels were significantly higher, 15%, compared with age-matched Caucasian American men.[25] It has been suggested that a difference in serum testosterone of 10% at this young age, if sustained, may explain the increased incidence of prostate cancer in African American men in later life.[26] Finally, in men with early-stage prostate cancer, soy isoflavones did not reduce either prostate specific antigen (PSA) or serum testosterone levels. Thus, the effectiveness of soy isoflavone in preventing prostate cancer is unknown.[27]

## Conclusion

Given the small number of studies evaluating the effect of soy on testosterone, no meaningful conclusion can be made regarding the effects of soy on testosterone. It is difficult to make comparisons regarding the different types and doses of soy products evaluated in the trials. Some studies suggest that soy consumption exerts small but possibly significant effects on testosterone. The difference in the effects on testosterone in the available studies may be dependent on the formulation consumed, the age of the subject population, both, or the ability to bind to the estrogen receptor. While the lowering of testosterone could be beneficial for the prevention of prostate cancer, it may be harmful for other health outcomes in men. Although the significance of soy effects in men is yet to be established, the evaluation of soy intake may be clinically important and should occur in men of all ages.

## References

1. Food labeling: health claims: soy protein and coronary heart disease. Food and Drug Administration, HHS: final rule: soy protein and coronary hear disease. *Fed Reg* 1999;64:57700-57733.

2. Anderson JW, Johnstone BM, Cook-Newell ME. Meta-analysis of the effects of soy protein intake on serum lipids. *N Engl J Med* 1995;333:276-282.

3. Erdman JW, Jr. Soy protein and cardiovascular disease: a statement for healthcare professionals from the nutrition committee of the AHA. *Circulation* 2000;102:2555-2559.

4. Reynolds K, Chin A, Lees KA, et al. A meta-analysis of the effect of soy protein supplementation on serum lipids. *Am J Cardiol* 2006;98:633-640.

5. Evidence Report/Technology Assessment No. 126, *Effects of Soy on Health Outcomes.* Agency for Healthcare Research and Quality 2005. Accessed at http://www.ahrq.gov/clinic/epc-sums/soysum.html

6. Erdman JW Jr, Badger TM, Lampe JW, et al. Not all soy products are created equal: caution needed in interpretation of research results. *J Nutr* 2004;134:1229S-1233S.

7. Goodin S, Shih WJ, Gallo M, et al. Effect of soy protein on testosterone levels. *Cancer Epidemiol Biomark Prev* 2007;16(12):2796.

8. Whitehead SA, Cross JE, Burden C, Lacey M. Acute and chronic effects of genistein, tyrphostin and lavendustin A on steroid synthesis in luteinized human granulose cells. *Hum Reprod* 2002;17:589-594.

9. Yi MA, Son HM, Lee JS, et al. Regulation of male sex hormone levels by soy isoflavones in rats. *Nutr Cancer* 2002;42:206-210.

10. Weber KS, Setchell KD, Stocco DM, Lephart ED. Dietary soy-phytoestrogens decrease testosterone levels and prostate weight without altering LH, prostate 5 alpha-reductase or testicular steroidogenic acute regulatory peptide levels in adult male Sprague-Dawley rats. *J Endocrinol* 2001;170:591-599.

11. Nagata C, Inaba S, Kawakami N, et al. Inverse association of soy product intake with serum androgen and estrogen concentrations in Japanese men. *Nutr Cancer* 2000;36:14-18.

12. Habito RC, Montalto J, Leslie J, Ball MJ. Effects of replacing meat with soyabean in the diet on sex hormone concentrations in healthy adult males. *Br J Nutr* 2000;84:557-563.

13. Nagata C, Takatsuka N, Shimizu H, et al. Effect of soymilk consumption on serum estrogen and androgen concentrations in Japanese men. *Cancer Epidemiol Biomark Prev* 2001;10:179-184.

14. Allen NE, Appleby PN, Davey GK, et al. Soy milk intake in relation to serum sex hormone levels in British men. *Nutr Cancer* 2001;41 (1&2): 41-46.

15. Mitchell JH, Cawood E, Kinigurgh D, et al. Effect of a phytoestrogen food supplement on reproductive health in normal males. *Clin Sci* 2001;100:613-618.

16. Teede HJ, Dalais FS, Kotsopoulos D, et al. Dietary soy has both beneficial and potentially adverse cardiovascular effects: a placebo-controlled study in men and postmenopausal women. *J Clin Endocrinol Metab* 2001;86(7):3053-60.

17. Gardner-Thorpe D, O'Hagen C, Young I, Lewis SJ. Dietary supplements of soya flour lower serum testosterone concentrations and improve markers of oxidative stress in men. *Eur J Clin Nutr* 2003;57:100-106.

18. Dillingham BL, McVeigh BL, Lampe JW, Duncan AM. Soy protein isolates of varying isoflavone content exert minor effects on serum reproductive hormones in healthy men. *J Nutr* 2005;135:584-591.

19. Goodin S, Shen F, Dave N, et al. Clinical and biological activity of soy protein powder supplementation in healthy male volunteers. *Cancer Epidemiol Biomarkers Prev* 2007: April 16(4):829-33.

20. Sharpe RM, Skakkebaek NE. Are estrogens involved in falling sperm counts and disorders of the male reproductive tract? *Lancet* 1993;341:1392-1395.

21. Bolona ER, Uraga MV, Haddad RM, et al. Testosterone use in men with sexual dysfunction: a systematic review and meta-analysis of randomized placebo-controlled trials. *Mayo Clin Proceed* 2007;82(1):20-28.

22. Isidori AM, Giannetta E, Pozza C, et al. Androgens, cardiovascular disease and osteoporosis. *J Endocrinol Invest* 2005:28(10 Suppl):73-79.

23. Khaw KT, Dowsett M, Folkerd E, et al. Endogenous testosterone and mortality due to all causes, cardiovascular disease, and cancer in men: European prospective investigation into cancer in Norfolk (EPIC-Norfolk) Prospective Population Study. *Circulation* 2007;116 (23):2694-701.

24. GA Barrett-Connor E, Bergstrom A. Low serum testosterone and mortality in older men. *J Clin Endocrinol Metab* 2008;93(1):68-75. Epub 2007 Oct 2.

25. Ross RK, Bernstein L, Judd H, et al. Serum testosterone in young black and white men. *J Natl Cancer Inst* 1986;76:45-48.

26. Ross RK, Henderson BE. Do diet and androgens alter prostate cancer risk via a common etiologic pathway? *J Natl Cancer Inst* 1994;86:252-254.

27. Kumar NB, Cantor, A, Allen K, et al. The specific role of isoflavones in reducing prostate cancer risk. *Prostate* 2004;59:141-147.

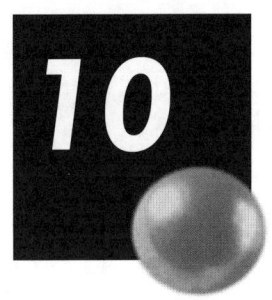

# Plan B Dosing for Plan B®: Alternative Dosing Strategies for Emergency Contraception with Levonorgestrel

*Laura B. Hansen*

## Background and Introduction

In 2001, 49% of pregnancies were unintended, meaning they were either mistimed or unwanted at the time of conception.[1] Of the 3.1 million unintended pregnancies, 44% ended in birth, 42% ended in abortion, and 14% ended in fetal loss. Furthermore, 48% of those unintended conceptions occurred during a month when contraception was used. Overall, 1 in 20 American women has an unintended pregnancy each year. When unintended pregnancies occur, serious and appreciable burdens can occur on women, children, and families. For example, mothers are at increased risk of maternal depression, anxiety, and a decline in psychological well-being; children born from unintended pregnancies are less likely to be breastfed or breastfed for a shorter duration and experience higher rates of child mortality and abuse compared to those from an intended pregnancy.[2] These unintended pregnancies and possible serious consequences could be potentially avoided if emergency contraception (EC) was administered in a timely manner. Situations considered appropriate for offering emergency contraception are listed in Table 10.1.[3]

Three emergency contraception strategies are currently employed in the United States: 1) insertion of the copper intrauterine device; 2) oral administration of a levonorgestrel-only regimen (Plan B®); and 3) oral administration of combined ethinyl estradiol (≥100 mcg per dose) with levonorgestrel/norgestrel, (≥0.5 mg levonorgestrel per dose) otherwise known as the Yuzpe regimen. The levonorgestrel-only regimen, Plan B, was approved by the Food and Drug Administration (FDA) in 1999; in 2006, it was switched from prescription to over-the-counter (OTC) status for women age 18 years and over. This EC regimen is often used, and pharmacists should be familiar with approved and alternative dosing strategies of the levonorgestrel-only regimen because physicians may instruct patients to use these alternative strategies. Several EC protocols encourage alternative dosing strategies.[4,5]

## FDA-Approved Dosing for Plan B®

The current FDA approved treatment for levonorgestrel used as EC is two doses of 0.75 mg; the first dose should be taken as soon as possible within 72 hours of unprotected intercourse,

**Table 10.1. Eligibility Criteria for Emergency Contraception[3]**

- No contraception used during intercourse
- Male or female condom slipped, broke, leaked, or was used incorrectly
- Incorrect use of diaphragm or cervical cap
- Missing combined oral contraceptives (COCs)
    - o    3 or more consecutive COCs with 30-35 mcg EE
    - o    2 or more consecutive COCs with ≤20 mcg EE
- ≥ 3 hr late for progestin-only pill
- ≥ 2 day late starting new vaginal ring cycle
- ≥ 2 day late starting new patch cycle
- > 14 days late getting a 3-month progestin-only contraceptive or date of previous injection unknown
- Couple erred in practicing coitus interruptus or periodic abstinence
- IUD partially or totally expelled or has been removed ≤ 7 days after last act of intercourse
- Woman exposed to possible teratogen (e.g., retinoic acid)

and the second dose should be taken 12 hours later. This regimen results in a 90% reduction in the risk of pregnancy.[6] In studies including more than 8,000 women, various doses of levonorgestrel-only EC reduced the risk of pregnancy by 60-94%.[7-12] It is important to note that effectiveness rates of EC compare the probability of pregnancy without treatment to that occurring with treatment. Therefore, with an EC effectiveness rate of 90% and with 80 pregnancies expected out of 1000 women without contraception, 10 pregnancies would be expected out of 1000 women if levonorgestrel EC was administered with this approved dosing regimen. Recent information indicates that these initial estimates of EC effectiveness may be too high, but EC should certainly still be offered because levonorgestrel EC is more effective in reducing the risk of pregnancy than no treatment at all.[13]

## Alternative Dosing Strategies for Plan B®

The 2005 American College of Obstetricians and Gynecologists (ACOG) practice bulletin on EC provides level A recommendations (based on good and consistent scientific evidence) for several different levonorgestrel EC dosing regimens.[14] Specifically, they recommend that the two 0.75 mg doses of the levonorgestrel regimen are equally effective if taken 12-24 hours apart and that the 1.5-mg levonorgestrel regimen can be taken as a single dose. As a level B recommendation (based on limited or inconsistent scientific evidence), ACOG recommended that EC should be made available to patients who request it up to 120 hours after unprotected intercourse. These three recommendations regarding alternative dosing strategies for levonorgestrel EC have also been supported by other major organizations (Table 10.2).

Pharmacists are actively involved in dispensing EC with and without a prescription. An accurate understanding of the evidence supporting these alternative dosing strategies is important, especially if pharmacists are asked to provide levonorgestrel EC in a regimen that is not approved by the FDA. The following three sections describe the best pharmacokinetic and patient outcome data for dosing levonorgestrel EC with alternative regimens.

## Compliance with Second Dose 12-24 Hours Later

Taking the second dose of levonorgestrel 0.75 mg can be justified through its pharmacologic properties as well as pharmacokinetic data. The half-life of levonorgestrel is long at $24.4 \pm 5.3$

**Table 10.2. Recommended Alternative Dosing Strategies from Major Organizations for the Levonorgestrel-only Emergency Contraception Regimen[22]**

| Organization | Take Second Dose 12-24 Hours After First | Take Both Tablets at Once (1.5 mg) | Offer Emergency Contraception ≤ 120 Hours After Intercourse |
|---|---|---|---|
| American Academy of Pediatrics | | X | |
| American College of Obstetricians and Gynecologists | X | X | X |
| Family Health International | | X | X |
| International Consortium for EC | | X | |
| Planned Parenthood | | X | X |
| World Health Organization | | X | X |

hours.[6] One study comparing the pharmacokinetics of levonorgestrel evaluated two 0.75 mg doses taken 12 hours apart, two 0.75 mg doses taken 24 hours apart, and a single 1.5 mg dose.[15] In this crossover trial including five women, levonorgestrel concentrations were measured at baseline, 1, 2, 4, 8, 12, 24, 36, 48, 60, 72, and 84 hours after each dose and then every 24 hours for 6 days. Mean time to maximum serum concentration (Tmax) was an estimated 1.5-1.8 hours after each of the two 0.75 mg doses and 2.6 hours after the single 1.5 mg dose. Peak plasma concentration (Cmax) was approximately 50% higher with the levonorgestrel single 1.5 mg dose compared with either 0.75 mg dose (p=0.03). Mean levonorgestrel concentrations at 48 hours were similar for all three treatment groups (6.2 and 7.4 nmol/L for the two 12- and 24-hour doses; 6.3 nmol/L for the single dose). The mean area under the curve (AUC) over the first 12 hours was significantly higher for the 1.5 mg single dose compared with the 12- and 24-hour 0.75 mg doses (282.4, 158.6, and 164.9 nmol/L, respectively; p=0.00014). It should be noted that the mean AUC over 24 hours did not differ for the two-dose regimens compared with the single dose regimen, but the total mean AUC over all days of observation was significantly higher for the single dose regimen than either two-dose regimens (p=0.0003). These data suggest that at least pharmacokinetically, a single dose of levonorgestrel 1.5 mg and a two-dose regimen of levonorgestrel 0.75 mg with the second dose taken 24 hours after the first, are at least comparable to the FDA-approved dose of levonorgestrel 0.75 mg with the second dose taken 12 hours after the first.

Few studies have directly compared the two doses of levonorgestrel 0.75 mg given 12 versus 24 hours apart. One open-label, blind observer trial involved 24 women randomized to one of three levonorgestrel treatment groups: a single 0.75 mg dose, two 0.75 mg doses taken 12 hours apart, and two 0.75 mg doses taken 24 hours apart.[16] Levonorgestrel concentrations were measured at baseline and at 0.5, 1, 1.5, 2, 2.5, 3, 3.5, 4, 5, 6, 8, 12, 24, and 36 hours after levonorgestrel was taken. Absorption, distribution, and elimination profiles were similar with all three treatments with no statistically significant differences in Tmax, Cmax, elimination rate constant, half-life, and AUC. The investigators found that even with the two 0.75 mg doses taken 24 hours apart, the levonorgestrel plasma concentrations were more than 10 times higher than the minimum concentrations needed for clinical effectiveness.[17]

Two well-designed studies have provided patient outcome data to support taking the second dose of levonorgestrel 0.75 mg 24 hours after the first dose. A World Health Organization (WHO) double-blind, randomized trial involving 1955 women from 21 centers worldwide showed indirect effectiveness of a second dose taken 24 hours after the first.[11] In this study, 574 women taking levonorgestrel 0.75 were instructed to take the second dose 12 hours after the first, but were considered "correct" users of the regimen if they took the second dose within 24 hours after the first dose. This group showed a prevented pregnancy fraction (effectiveness) of 89% (5/574 pregnancies) and therefore indicated that two doses of levonorgestrel 0.75 mg taken up to 24 hours apart may be effective.

A double-blind, randomized trial of 2071 women from five sites in China compared the effectiveness of two doses of levonorgestrel 0.75 mg given at either a 12- or 24-hour interval, with treatment offered up to 120 hours after unprotected intercourse.[9] The primary outcome of pregnancy was analyzed in 2018 women with 998 in the 12-hour group and 1020 in the 24-hour group. The crude pregnancy rates were 2.0% in the 12-hour group (95% CI 1.19-2.99) and 1.9% in the 24-hour group (95% CI 1.17-2.94). With 20 pregnancies in each group, the proportion of prevented pregnancies was 75% in the 12-hour group (95% CI 59.0-83.7) and 72% in the 24-hour group (95% CI 56.7-82.7). Furthermore, efficacy was not significantly different when treatment was given within 72 hours versus up to 120 hours after unprotected intercourse. These data support two doses of levonorgestrel 0.75 mg given 12- or 24-hours apart as well as starting therapy up to 120 hours after unprotected intercourse.

## Double Up with Two Tablets at Once

In addition to the study described earlier,[15] pharmacokinetic evidence has demonstrated effective levonorgestrel plasma concentrations when 1.5 mg is given in a single dose. Thirty healthy women in the periovulatory phase of their menstrual cycle were prospectively randomized to receive oral placebo (five women), oral levonorgestrel 1.5 mg single dose (13 women), or vaginal levonorgestrel 1.5 mg single dose (12 women).[18] Primary outcome measures were levonorgestrel concentrations in the plasma (n=30) and the endometrial tissue (n=11). Mean peak concentrations were achieved sooner with the oral regimen (1-4 versus 6-8 hours after oral versus vaginal administration, $p<0.05$) and were 6 times higher ($C_{max}$ 64.0 versus 10.0 nmol/L, $p<0.05$). Although mean ± SD concentrations were significantly higher for oral administration at 24 hours, concentrations were similar in both groups at 168 hours and above minimal effective concentration. This study supports a single dose of oral (or vaginal) levonorgestrel 1.5 mg for emergency contraception based on pharmacokinetic information.

Patient outcome data for providing levonorgestrel 1.5 mg as a single dose was demonstrated in a prospective, double-blind trial comparing safety and efficacy in 1118 Nigerian women seeking EC within 72 hours of unprotected sexual intercourse.[7] In this study, 545 women were randomized to two doses of levonorgestrel 0.75 mg taken 12 hours apart, and 573 women were randomized to a single dose of levonorgestrel 1.5 mg. Efficacy was measured by evaluation of pregnancy rates through crude relative risk and prevention of expected pregnancies. Crude pregnancy rates were not statistically significantly different and reported as 1.28% (7/545) from the two-dose group and 0.69% (4/573) from the single-dose group (RR 0.71, 95% CI 0.32-1.55, $p>0.05$). However, the estimated effectiveness rate for all conceptions was higher in the single-dose group compared with the two-dose group (93.9% versus 88.6%, $p<0.05$). In terms of safety, women in the two-dose group had significantly less headache and breast tenderness ($p<0.05$), but more vomiting, dizziness, and lower abdominal pain than that of the single-dose group.

Another multicenter, double-blind trial from the WHO, demonstrated efficacy with the single- and two-dose levonorgestrel regimens.[8] This study involved 4071 women from 10 different countries who were requesting emergency contraception within 120 hours of unprotected sexual intercourse. Patients were randomized to a single dose of levonorgestrel 1.5 mg (n=1356), two doses of levonorgestrel 0.75 mg taken 12 hours apart (n=1356), or a single dose of mifepristone 10 mg (n=1059), which is a regimen not approved for EC in the United States but is often used in other countries. Results of the primary outcome, unintended pregnancy, indicated no significant differences between the two levonorgestrel dosing strategies. The crude rates of pregnancy were 1.47% (20/1356) in the single-dose group and 1.77% (24/1356) in the two-dose group. The estimated reduction in expected pregnancy was 82% (95% CI 70.9-88.7) in the single-dose group and 77% (95% CI 64.9-85.4) in the two-dose group and did not differ between groups (0.80, 95% CI 0.42-1.51). Adverse effect rates for nausea and vomiting were similar in both groups. Therefore, efficacy and tolerability were similar with both the 1.5 mg single-dose and the 0.75 mg two-dose levonorgestrel strategies.

Another study comparing only the levonorgestrel 1.5 mg single-dose and mifepristone 10 mg single dose regimens indicated that levonorgestrel 1.5 mg is effective as a single dose in reducing expected pregnancy rates.[12] Additionally, levonorgestrel is increasingly being marketed internationally as a single-dose formulation (one 1.5 mg tablet) rather than a two-dose formulation (two 0.75 mg tablets taken 12 hours apart).[13]

## Extend the Time Frame for Offering Plan B®

Several studies have indicated that the levonorgestrel regimen is more effective the closer the dosing is to the time of unprotected or underprotected intercourse.[8,10,11] However, a few studies have not observed this timed effect with levonorgestrel, although sample sizes were small.[9,10,12,19] Initial studies included only women who used the levonorgestrel regimen within 72 hours of intercourse and consequently the package insert for Plan B® and older guidelines advise use only within that time frame.[6]

More recent studies show that EC remains moderately effective if started between 72 to 120 hours, and a few studies evaluating the administration of levonorgestrel in this extended time frame have been described previously.[8,9] Most trials assessing the effectiveness of EC from 72 to 120 hours have been done with the combined (estrogen-progestin) oral contraceptive pills. In a study of 131 women receiving EC within 72 hours compared with 169 women receiving EC within 72 to 120 hours, the effectiveness rate was 87-90% for the < 72-hour group and 72-87% for the 72- to 120-hour group.[20] In both groups, it was demonstrated that EC significantly reduced the risk of pregnancy ($p<0.05$) compared with the expected pregnancy rate. Addtionally, investigators performing an observational study with small power suggested that the 72-hour cutoff for EC was "needlessly restrictive."[21] Overall, EC should be made available to patients who request it up to 120 hours after intercourse. There are currently no data evaluating EC effectiveness when starting EC more than 120 hours after unprotected or underprotected intercourse.

# Conclusion

Pharmacists have an active role in the dispensing and counseling of levonorgestrel EC. They need to be informed of alternative dosing strategies with this regimen because they may be asked to provide it to patients in a manner that is not approved by the FDA. Several major organizations and women's health groups support these alternative regimens based on evidence and opportunity for improved adherence and access to EC. In summary, there can be a plan A through E:

Plan A – All goes well with protection during sexual intercourse.

Plan B – Broken condom, birth control pills are missed, or other event results in a need for levonorgestrel EC; 0.75 mg for the first dose given within 72 hours and 0.75 mg for the second dose given 12 hours later.

Plan C – Compliance with the second levonorgestrel dose can occur 12-24 hours after first dose.

Plan D – Doubling up by taking both levonorgestrel tablets at once is effective.

Plan E – Extending the time frame up to 120 hours for starting EC is appropriate.

# References

1. Finer LB, Henshaw SK. Disparities in rates of unintended pregnancy in the United States, 1994 and 2001. *Perspect Sex Reprod Health* 2006;38:90-96.

2. Gipson JD, Koenig MA, Hindin MJ. The effects of unintended pregnancy on infant, child, and parental health: a review of the literature. *Stud Fam Plan* 2008;39:18-38.

3. Stewart F, Trussell J, Van Look PFA. Emergency contraception. In Hatcher RA, Trussell J, Nelson AL, Cates W, Stewart FH, Kowal D, eds. *Contraceptive Technology.* 19th ed. New York: Ardent Media Inc.; 2007:87-116.

4. Planned Parenthood. Emergency Contraception (Morning After Pill). Available at: http://www.plannedparenthood.org/health-topics/emergency-contraception-morning-after-pill-4363.htm#use. Accessed June 5, 2008.

5. California state emergency contraception drug therapy collaborative agreement protocol. Available at: http://www.pharmacyaccess.org/pdfs/ECCollabProtocol.pdf Accessed June 5, 2008.

6. Plan B [package insert]. Pomona, NY: DuraMed Pharmaceuticals; 2006.

7. Arowojolu AO, Okewole IA, Adekunle AO. Comparative evaluation of the effectiveness and safety of two regimens of levonorgestrel for emergency contraception in Nigerians [published erratum appears in Contraception 2003;67:165]. *Contraception* 2002;66:269-273.

8. von Hertzen H, Piaggio G, Ding J, et al. Low dose mifepristone and two regimens of levonorgestrel for emergency contraception: a WHO multicentre randomised trial. *Lancet* 2002;360:1803-1810.

9. Ngai SW, Fan S, Li S, et al. A randomized trial to compare 24 h versus 12 h double dose regimen of levonorgestrel for emergency contraception. *Hum Reprod* 2005;20:307-311.

10. Ho PC, Kwan MS. A prospective randomized comparison of levonorgestrel with the Yuzpe regimen in post-coital contraception. *Hum Reprod* 1993;8:389-392.

11. Task Force on Postovulatory Methods of Fertility Regulation. Randomised controlled trial of levonorgestrel versus the Yuzpe regimen of combined oral contraceptives for emergency contraception. *Lancet* 1998;352:428-33.

12. Hamoda H, Ashok PW, Stalder C, et al. A randomized trial of mifepristone (10 mg) and levonorgestrel for emergency contraception. *Obstet Gynecol* 2004;104:1307-13.

13. Trussell J, Raymond EG. Emergency contraception: a last chance to prevent unintended pregnancy. Available at: http://ec.princeton.edu/questions/ec-review.pdf. Accessed June 4, 2008.

14. American College of Obstetricians and Gynecologists. ACOG practice bulletin. Clinical management guidelines for obstetrician-gynecologists, no. 69, December 2005 (replaces practice bulletin no. 25, March 2001): emergency contraception. *Obstet Gynecol* 2005;106:1443-1452.

15. Johansson E, Brache V, Alvarez F, et al. Pharmacokinetic study of different dosing regimens of levonorgestrel for emergency contraception in healthy women. *Hum Reprod* 2002;17:1472-1476.

16. Tremblay D, Gainer E, Ulmann A. The pharmacokinetics of 750 μg levonorgestrel following administration of one single dose or two doses at 12- or 24-h interval. *Contraception* 2001;64:327-331.

17. Nilsson CG, Lahteenmaki P, Luukkainen T. Patterns of ovulation and bleeding with a low levonorgestrel-releasing intrauterine device. *Contraception* 1980;21:155-164.

18. Devoto L, Fuentes A, Palomino A, et al. Pharmacokinetics and endometrial tissue levels of levonorgestrel after administration of a single 1.5-mg dose by the oral and vaginal route. *Fertil Steril* 2005;84:46-51.

19. Wu S, Wang C, Wang Y, et al. A randomized, double-blind, multicenter study on comparing levonorgestrel and mifepristone for emergency contraception. *J Reprod Med* 1999;8(suppl 1):43-46.

20. Rodrigues I, Grou F, Joly J. Effectiveness of emergency contraceptive pills between 72 and 120 hours after unprotected sexual intercourse. *Am J Obstet Gynecol* 2001;184:531-537.

21. Ellertson C, Evans M, Ferden S, et al. Extending the time limit for starting the Yuzpe regimen of emergency contraception to 120 hours. *Obstet Gynecol* 2003;1168-1171.

22. Hansen LB, Saseen JS, Teal SB. Levonorgestrel-only dosing strategies for emergency contraception. *Pharmacotherapy* 2007;27:278-284.

# Warfarin and Cotrimoxazole: Averting Disaster

*Todd R. Marcy*

## Introduction

Warfarin is an anticoagulant drug used for the prevention and treatment of thromboembolic disorders, such as venous thromboembolism and cardioembolic stroke.[1] Patients with a history of deep vein thrombosis, pulmonary embolism, atrial fibrillation, or prosthetic heart valves are commonly prescribed warfarin for periods ranging from 3 months to lifelong. The medical community has a rich experience with warfarin. It has been used since the early 1950s.[2]

Vitamin K is a key cofactor in the synthesis of functional coagulation factors II, VII, IX, and X. Warfarin exerts its effect by inhibition of the hepatic cyclic interconversion of vitamin K and its epoxide, thereby preventing the recycling of vitamin K and reducing production of fully functional coagulation factors.[1,2,3] The onset of action is dependent upon the metabolism of the vitamin K-dependant clotting factors present prior to warfarin initiation. These factors must be metabolized prior to the onset of warfarin's effect, as warfarin has no activity against functional clotting factors. Factor II has the longest half-life, approximately 60-72 hours.[3]

Warfarin is a racemic mixture of S and R isomers. S-warfarin is approximately 3-5 times more potent than R-warfarin. S- and R-warfarin are metabolized by different cytochrome P450 enzymes. S-warfarin is metabolized predominantly by 2C9 and R-warfarin by 1A2, 2C19, and 3A4.[2] Warfarin is approximately 99% protein-bound.[1]

The effect of warfarin is measured by the International Normalized Ratio (INR). A healthy individual not treated with warfarin is expected to have an INR value near 1.0. The anticoagulation status increases as the INR increases. Usual target INR ranges for patients treated with warfarin are 2.0-3.0 or 2.5-3.5, depending upon the indication. This range may be adjusted based on a patient's variance from usual in regards to thromboembolic or hemorrhagic risk.

There are a number of inherited, acquired, and environmental factors that significantly influence the degree to which warfarin impacts a patient's INR. These include, but are not limited to: genetic variations in CYP 2C9 (altered S-warfarin metabolism) and vitamin K epoxide reductase complex 1(VKCORC1) (altered response to warfarin),[1] a variety of acute or chronic illnesses, fluctuations in dietary vitamin K intake, and a litany of drug interactions.[4] These and other factors may change over time, resulting in fluctuations of INR values and the need for regular INR monitoring, at least every 4 weeks.

The consequences of out-of-range INR values are increasing risk of thromboembolism (with sub-therapeutic INR values) or significant hemorrhage (with supra-therapeutic INR values).

In one study, patients treated with warfarin for atrial fibrillation who had poor anticoagulation control (as measured by the percent time a patient's INR is in therapeutic range) had increased rates of ischemic events. Patients in the lowest tertile of time in therapeutic range had stroke or systemic embolism rates that were nearly twice as high as patients in the top tertile of the category (p=0.02).[5]

There are clear associations between intensity of anticoagulant effect and risk of major bleeding. For example, one case-control study found a doubling in the risk of intracerebral hemorrhage with each increase of approximately 1.0 in the INR.[6] The consequences of major bleeding can include death, disability, hospital admission, and transfusions.

Cotrimoxazole (also known as sulfamethoxazole/trimethoprim, Bactrim®, and Septra®) is a combination antibiotic agent with a broad spectrum of antimicrobial activity commonly used in the treatment of a variety of infections. For example, cotrimoxazole can be used to treat some infections of the urinary, respiratory, and gastrointestinal systems.[7] Sulfamethoxazole is about 70% protein bound, and trimethoprim is about 44% protein bound.[8] Sulfamethoxazole is hepatically metabolized predominantly through $N_4$-acetylation. The glucuronide conjugate has also been identified.[8]

There is a well-documented drug interaction between warfarin and cotrimoxizole. If not appropriately managed, the usual effect is a notable increase in the INR and subsequent increased risk of a significant hemorrhagic event. If the interaction is identified, but the warfarin dose is too aggressively reduced, then the INR may become sub-therapeutic thereby increasing thromboembolic risk. Although the effect is documented, specific data and recommendations regarding the management of this interaction are lacking.

## Mechanisms of Drug Interactions with Warfarin

There are a litany of drugs that when co-administered with warfarin increase hemorrhagic or thromboembolic risk. The mechanisms for these interactions are many and are contributed to by the narrow therapeutic window of warfarin. Some interactions directly influence warfarin availability and others increase hemorrhagic or thromboembolic risk independent of warfarin. Mechanisms of interaction can be categorized into drugs that alter the availability of free warfarin in vivo, drugs that alter the availability or cyclic interconversion of hepatic vitamin K,[3] drugs that alter the metabolism of coagulation factors, and drugs that otherwise alter a patient's hemorrhagic or thromboembolic risk (Table 11.1).

Mechanisms of interactions that alter the availability of warfarin include the following: inhibition or induction of S-warfarin metabolism, inhibition or induction of R-warfarin metabolism, inhibition of warfarin absorption, and displacement of warfarin from plasma proteins.

## Warfarin-Cotrimoxazole Interaction

The drug interaction between warfarin and cotrimoxazole is well documented in case reports,[13-17] systematic reviews,[4] and accepted practice guidelines.[3] The mechanism of the interaction is thought to be inhibition of S-warfarin metabolism through CYP 2C9 and displacement of

## Table 11.1. Warfarin Drug–Drug Interaction Summary

| Category | Mechanism | Potential Effect | Example |
|---|---|---|---|
| Warfarin availability | Inhibition of S-warfarin metabolism | ↑ INR | Metronidazole[3] |
| | Inihibition of R-warfarin metabolism | ↑ INR (usually modest) | Omeprazole[3] |
| | Displacemnt of warfarin from plasma proteins | ↑ INR | Valproate[2] |
| | Inhibition of warfarin absorption | ↓ INR | Cholestyramine[2] |
| | Induction of S- and/or R- warfarin metabolism | ↓ INR | Carbamazepine[2,9] |
| Vitamin K availability | Reduced absoprtion of dietary vitamin K | ↑ INR | Orlistat[10] |
| | Inhibition of cyclic interconversion of vitamin K | ↑ INR | Cephalosporins[2,3] |
| | Elimination of vitamin K-producing gut flora | ↑ INR | Broad spectrum antibiotics[2,3] |
| Coagulation pathway changes | Increase metabolism of coagulation factors | ↑ INR | Levothyroxine[2] |
| | Increase synthesis of coagulation factors | ↓ or ↔ INR | Oral contraceptive hormones[11] |
| | Acquired activated protein C resistance | ↔ INR | Third generation oral contraceptives [12] |
| Other changes in hemorrhagic risk | Impairment of prostaglandin lining of the GI-tract | ↔ INR | NSAIDS |
| | Platelet inhibition | ↔ INR | Clopidogrel[2] |

warfarin from protein binding sites by cotrimoxazole.[14,15]   The clinical result is an increased availability of free warfarin and an enhanced anticoagulation effect, reflected by an elevated INR.   Factors associated with the infection for which cotrimoxazole is used may also influence the INR.   These may include: fever, dietary changes, warfarin adherence, diarrhea, or emesis.

The magnitude of the increase in the INR is variable, but often significant.   A retrospective study evaluated 16 outpatients in a Veteran's Affairs Medical Center with stable warfarin therapy who were initiated on cotrimoxazole without warfarin dose adjustment.[18]   The mean follow-up after initiation was 6 days, with a mean change in the INR of 1.76.   Sixty-nine percent of patients had a follow-up INR that was supra-therapeutic (31% were therefore not supra-thera-peutic), 56% had an INR increase of 1.0 or more, 38% had an INR increase of 2.0 or more, 44% had an absolute INR of 4.0 or higher, and 31% had an absolute INR of 5.0 or higher. It is evident from this data that there is significant patient–patient variability in the degree to which cotrimoxazole effects the INR, but that it is often a clinically significant increase.   This is consistent with anecdotal observations caring for patients in an anticoagulation clinic.

The consequences of this interaction can be severe.   Data regarding the incidence of signifi-cant hemorrhagic events due to this interaction have not been reported.   However,   documented cases of hospitalizations for such events has been reported in the literature.[15-17]

## Clinical Experience with the Interaction

The University of Oklahoma College of Pharmacy operates an anticoagulation clinic in which pharmacists manage warfarin therapy.   Patients are referred to our outpatient service from their primary care physician or specialist.   Patients are followed longitudinally and evaluated at intervals of no more than 4 weeks.   Patients are assessed for hemorrhagic or thromboembolic events and for factors potentially influencing their INR (such as acute infection and new medications). Warfarin dose adjustments are made as appropriate.

Patients in the service are consistently educated about warfarin drug interactions and encour-aged to contact clinic personnel prior to initiation of any new prescription or over-the-counter medication. Medication histories are performed at each clinic visit to evaluate any changes to drug therapy not reported by the patient since the last visit. Reporting of cotrimoxazole therapy has occurred both prior to initiation (as directed) and at regularly scheduled follow-up visits after initiation of cotrimoxazole therapy.

Barriers to appropriate management of this interaction include:  prescriber unawareness of the interaction, prescriber unawareness of warfarin therapy, patient failure to report cotri-moxazole initiation to the anticoagulation clinic, pharmacy failure to identify or act upon the interaction at the point of filling cotrimoxazole prescription, and anticoagulation clinic failure to identify the new medication.

Consistent with the study by Glasheen,[18] INR response following cotrimoxazole use in this population is variable.   Most patients have an INR increase that results in a supra-therapeu-tic INR value.   The magnitude of increase is variable, but the INR frequently surpasses 5.0. However, cases have been observed in which a therapeutic INR has been maintained without empiric changes to warfarin therapy.

There are a number of possible explanations for the considerable inter-patient variability that exists with the warfarin–cotrimoxazole interaction.   There is inter-patient variability in the likely mechanisms of interaction, namely the degree of inhibition of CYP 2C9 and the availability for warfarin protein-binding displacement. Factors potentially influencing a patient's INR beyond the cotrimoxazole–warfarin interaction, particularly in patients with an infectious illness have been described.

Planned co-administration of warfarin and cotrimoxazole is imprecise. Extreme INR values can usually be avoided with empiric warfarin dose reductions and careful monitoring. However, maintenance of a therapeutic INR throughout cotrimoxazole therapy is difficult. Further, patient adherence to increased monitoring when they are suffering from an infectious illness is variable.

Patients will sometimes be prescribed chronic cotrimoxazole therapy for prophylaxis from urinary tract infections or pneumocystis carinii pneumonia.[19] When patients prescribed warfarin are initiated on chronic cotrimoxazole therapy, the effect on the INR is similar to the transient use of the antibiotic. However, the effect is maintained over the duration of cotrimoxazole use. If the patient maintains excellent adherence to both cotrimoxazole and warfarin, a new warfarin maintenance dose can usually be identified with careful monitoring.

## Recommended Management

Management of the cotrimoxazole–warfarin interaction is complicated by inter-patient variability in INR response when cotrimoxazole is added. Therefore, when the interaction is identified, the prescriber should be contacted to discuss therapeutic alternatives to cotrimoxazole therapy.

There are circumstances under which cotrimoxazole is the optimal anti-infective agent, intentional management of the interaction is an option, and the increase in hemorrhagic and thromboembolic risk may be worth the benefit provided by cotrimoxazole in an individual patient. This may be particularly true in patients at less than the highest risk for a hemorrhagic or thromboembolic event if their INR were to become modestly out-of-range.

There are no accepted consensus recommendations for the management of this interaction. The University of Oklahoma College of Pharmacy Anticoagulation service employs a patient-specific approach to managing this interaction. The prescriber is contacted to confirm the appropriateness of the use of cotrimoxazole. If the decision to use this agent is confirmed, the patient's thromboembolic and hemorrhagic risks are assessed. Patients at the highest risk can be considered for interruption of warfarin therapy and initiation of an alternative anticoagulant agent. This may be an appropriate consideration for patients who have had a thromboembolic or hemorrhagic event with an INR value that was modestly out-of-range. In this circumstance, a low molecular weight heparin (LMWH) could be used until the cotrimoxazole therapy is complete. Warfarin would be reinitiated and LMWH would be continued until the INR has returned to a therapeutic level. This option may also be selected for patients in whom close INR monitoring is inaccessible.

When the decision is made to use warfarin and cotrimoxazole concomitantly, patient records are reviewed for previous concurrent use of the agents. The warfarin dose reduction is made based on the patient's previous response and assessed thromboembolic and hemorrhagic risk. The patient's INR and warfarin dose is reassessed every 1 to 3 days until cotrimoxazole therapy is complete.

## Table 11.2. Summary of Recommendations for Managing Warfarin–Cotrimoxazole Interaction

1. Contact prescribing physician to assess appropriateness of an alternative antibiotic.

   a. If cotrimoxazole is required, assess hemorrhagic and thromboembolic risk.

   b. Assess accessibility of close INR monitoring.

2. If hemorrhagic or thromboembolic risk are unacceptably high or accessibility to close INR monitoring is poor, consider bridging with a low-molecular weight heparin (LMWH) product. If LMWH chosen, discontinue warfarin until cotrimoxazole therapy is complete.

3. If warfarin is selected, review record to identify history of concomitant warfarin–cotrimoxazole use. Base warfarin empiric dose reduction on this history and monitor every 1-3 days.

4. If there is no history of concomitant use, empirically lower warfarin dose 20-40% based on assessed relative hemorrhagic and thromboembolic risk. Monitor every 1-3 days.

When managing the interaction for the first time in an individual patient, empiric dose reductions should be based on assessed relative risks. A standard reduction in warfarin dosing of about 30% is generally appropriate. For patients at high thromboembolic risk relative to hemorrhagic risk, an empiric warfarin dose reduction of 20-30% is reasonable. For patients at higher relative hemorrhagic risk, an empiric warfarin dose reduction of 30-40% is reasonable. The INR and warfarin dosing should be reassessed every 1 to 3 days until cotrimoxazole therapy is complete.

Once cotrimoxazole is complete, assess the INR value. If it is therapeutic, resume the previous warfarin maintenance dose. If the INR is out-of-range, temporarily (i.e., 1-2 days) adjust the warfarin dose based on the value, then resume the previous maintenance warfarin dose. See Table 11.2 for a summary of the recommended management of the interaction.

## Case Study

A case example may be helpful to illustrate this approach. CP is a 59-year-old Caucasian man with a St. Jude mechanical heart valve in the mitral position. His past relevant medical history includes: left ventricular (LV) dysfunction (ejection fraction 25%) and hypertension (currently well controlled). He has no history of stroke, hemorrhagic complications, renal dysfunction, or diabetes. He has had a therapeutic INR each month for the last 6 months with a warfarin dose of 5 mg daily (35 mg per week). His target INR range is 2.5–3.5, and it is 3.0 today. He was prescribed a 7-day course of twice daily cotrimoxazole. This is his first course of cotrimoxazole while prescribed warfarin therapy. After confirmation with the prescriber that cotrimoxazole use is necessary, the clinical pharmacist assesses CP's risks. He is at relatively low risk for a hemorrhagic event (risk includes anticoagulation with warfarin and hypertension). Thromboembolic risks include the mechanical heart valve in the mitral position with LV dysfunction and hypertension. Based on the patient's risk, the pharmacist values prevention of a thromboembolic event over that of a hemorrhagic one because a thromboembolic event with a modestly sub-therapeutic INR is more likely than a hemorrhagic event with a modestly supra-therapeutic INR. The pharmacist plans a warfarin dose reduction of 20-30%. He instructs the patient to take 2.5 mg today and 5 mg tomorrow and to follow up on the third day prior to warfarin dosing. This represents a 25% reduction in his usual dose (7.5 mg as opposed to usual 10 mg over a 2-day period). Subsequent adjustments will be made following evaluation of his response to cotrimoxazole on his adjusted warfarin dose.

## Conclusion

Warfarin is an anticoagulant agent with a narrow therapeutic window. Hemorrhagic and thromboembolic risk increases as the distance an INR increases outside of target range. There is a significant drug interaction between warfarin and cotrimoxazole that when left unmanaged, usually results in an increase in the INR beyond therapeutic levels. However, there is considerable patient–patient variability in response to this interaction. It is optimal to avoid this interaction and use an alternative antibiotic agent in place of cotrimoxazole. If necessary, the interaction can be managed in appropriate patients, with empiric warfarin dose reductions and careful monitoring.

## References

1. Package insert. Coumadin (warfarin sodium tablets, USP). Princeton, NJ: Bristol-Myers Squibb Co., August 2007.
2. Majerus PW, Tollefsen DM. Blood coagulation and anticoagulant, thrombolytic, and antiplatelet drugs. In: Brunton LL, Lazo JS, Parker KL, eds. Goodman & Gillman's: The Pharmacological Basis of Therapeutics. 11th ed. New York: McGraw-Hill, 2006:1467-88.
3. Ansell J, Hirsh J, Poller L, et al. The pharmacology and management of the vitamin K antagonists. *CHEST* 2004;126:204S-33S.
4. Holbrook AM, Pereira JA, Labiris R, et al. Systematic overview of warfarin and its drug and food interactions. *Arch Intern Med* 2005;165:1095-106.
5. White HD, Gruber M, Feyzi J, et al. Comparison of outcomes among patients randomized to warfarin therapy according to anticoagulation control. *Arch Intern Med* 2007;167:239-45.
6. Hylek EM, Singer DE. Risk factors for intracranial hemorrhage in outpatients taking warfarin. *Ann Intern Med* 1994;120:897-902.

7. Petri, WA. Sulfonamides, trimethoprim-sulfamethoxazole, quinolones, and agents for urinary track infections. In: Brunton LL, Lazo JS, Parker KL, eds. Goodman & Gillman's: The Pharmacological Basis of Therapeutics. 11th ed. New York: McGraw-Hill, 2006:1111-26.

8. Package insert. Bactrim (sulfamethoxazole and trimethoprim double strength). Philadelphia: AR Scientific, March 2005.

9. McNamara JO. Pharmacotherapy of the epilepsies. In: Brunton LL, Lazo JS, Parker KL, eds. Goodman & Gillman's: The Pharmacological Basis of Therapeutics. 11th ed. New York: McGraw-Hill, 2006:501-25.

10. MacWalters RS, Fraser HW, Armstrong KM. Orlistat enhances warfarin effect. *Ann Pharmacother* 2003;37:510-2.

11. Battaglioli T, Martinelli I. Hormone therapy and thromboembolic disease. Curr Opin Hematol. 2007;14:488-93.

12. Tans G, Curvers J, Middeldorp S, et al. A randomized cross-over study on the effects of levonorgestrel- and desogestrel-containing oral contraceptives on the anticoagulant pathways. *Thromb Haemost* 2000;84:15-21.

13. Cook DE, Ponte CD. Suspected trimethoprim/sulfamethoxazole-induced hypoprothrominemia. *J Fam Pract* 1994;39:589-91.

14. O'Reilly RA. Stereoselective interaction of trimethoprim-sulfamethoxazole with the separated enantiomorphs of racemic warfarin in man. *N Engl J Med* 1980;302:33-5.

15. Richmond RG, Sawyer WT, Aiello PD, et al. Extreme warfarin intoxication secondary to possible covert drug ingestion. *Drug Intell Clin Pharm* 1988;22:696-9.

16. Chaffin CC, Ritter BA, James A, et al. Hospital admission due to warfarin potentiation by TMP-SMX. *Nurse Pract* 2000;25:73-5.

17. Erichsen C, Sondenaa K, Soreide J, et al. Spontaneous liver hematomas induced by anti-coagulation therapy: a case report and review of the literature. *Hepato-Gastroenterol* 1993;40:402-6.

18. Glasheen JJ, Fugit RV, Prochazka AV. The risk of overanticoagulation with antibiotic use in outpatients on stable warfarin regimens. *J Gen Intern Med* 2005;20:653-6.

19. CDC. USPHS/IDSA Guidelines for preventing opportunistic infections among HIV-infected persons. *MMWR* 2002;51(No. RR08):1-46.

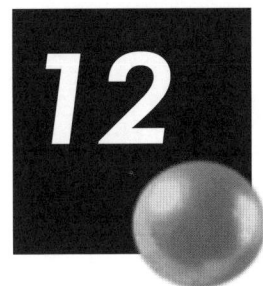

# 12 Celiac Disease: Dangers of Gluten in Medications

*Robert A. Mangione*

## Background and Introduction

Celiac disease (at times referred to as celiac sprue) is a chronic autoimmune disorder that is caused by a genetic intolerance to gluten.[1] Gluten, which is a storage protein, is the component of bread and other baked goods that makes them doughy and elastic.[2] It is also found in many other food products and in medications. While the term "gluten" actually refers to the entire protein component of wheat, the proteins that cannot be tolerated by (and cause intestinal damage and other symptoms in) celiac disease patients are gliadins (wheat) as well as related proteins hordeins (barley) and secalins (rye).[3] Therefore, patients with this disease must not ingest wheat, barley, or rye.

Although it was originally reported to be a pediatric syndrome characterized by diarrhea, steatorrhea, and weight loss it is now recognized that celiac disease may be diagnosed in patients of varied ages and that it may cause a variety of symptoms. The presence of celiac disease must continue to be considered in children; however, adult presentations are now more common and diagnoses in patients with nondiarrheal symptoms, referred to as silent or atypical presentations, are becoming more frequent.[1,4] Celiac disease, like other autoimmune diseases, is more frequently diagnosed in women than in men. Although the gastrointestinal system is the primary site of injury, it is very important to recognize that celiac disease is a multisystem disease.[1,3]

Recent findings in the United States suggest that the prevalence of celiac disease is much greater than originally thought (as many as 3 million Americans or approximately 1 percent of the United States population may be affected).[4] Educational and advocacy efforts have helped to increase the rate of diagnosis; however, the disease is still widely overlooked. It is currently estimated that 97 percent of celiac disease patients have not been diagnosed, leading some experts to refer to celiac disease as a "hidden epidemic."[3] There is a great need to improve the diagnosis rate of this disease and to avoid misdiagnosing these patients with other ailments[2] (Table 12.1). Poor diet compliance and undiagnosed disease are associated with increased morbidity and mortality.[5,6] Pharmacists can play an important role in identifying patients who may have celiac disease, referring these patients for proper evaluation, and assisting with the management of this disease.

## Table 12.1. Some Common Misdiagnoses Prior to Confirmation of Celiac Disease[2]

### Gastrointestinal

| | |
|---|---|
| Irritable bowel syndrome | Ulcers |
| Inflammatory bowel disease | Gastroesophageal reflux disease |
| Gallbladder disease | Amoebae/parasitic infection |
| Viral gastroenteritis | "Spastic colon" |
| Lactose intolerance | Colitis |

### Other

| | |
|---|---|
| Cystic fibrosis | Allergies |
| Psychological dysfunction | Chronic fatigue syndrome |

## Table 12.2. Selected Reported Clinical Manifestations of Celiac Disease[7]

### Typical symptoms

| | |
|---|---|
| Chronic diarrhea | Anorexia |
| Failure to thrive | Abdominal distension |

### Atypical symptoms related to malabsorption

| | |
|---|---|
| Iron deficiency anemia | Recurrent abortions |
| Short stature | Bloating |
| Osteopenia | Recurrent abdominal pain |

### Atypical symptoms not related to malabsorption

| | |
|---|---|
| Dental enamel hypoplasia | Persistent aphthous stomatitis |
| Ataxia | Hypertransaminasemia |
| Alopecia | Vasculitis |
| Polyneuropathy | Infertility |
| Dermatitis herpetiformis | |

# Diagnosis of Celiac Disease

A critically important initial step in making the diagnosis of celiac disease is for clinicians to understand this disease and to recognize its many possible symptoms[5,7] (Table 12.2 ). Only 3 percent of patients with celiac disease have been diagnosed, therefore, pharmacists can play a critical role in identifying patients who may benefit from a diagnostic evaluation.

A duodenal biopsy that demonstrates the characteristic findings of intraepithelial lymphocytes, crypt hyperplasia and villous atrophy, and a positive response to a gluten-free diet are required to confirm a diagnosis.[1] Serological tests are useful adjunctive diagnostic tools; in fact, most celiac disease patients are currently being identified due to testing for serologic markers for the disease.[8] These tests are non-invasive and facilitate screening of large populations.[7, 9]

Although serologic tests for the presence of gliadin antibodies have been available for over 30 years, testing for endomysial IgA antibodies or anti-tissue transglutaminase antibodies is now generally preferred due to the greater sensitivity and specificity of these tests.[8] Testing for anti-tissue transglutaminase antibodies provides clinicians with an automated enzyme linked immunosorbent assay (ELISA) serologic test.[10]

# Management of Celiac Disease

Expert participants at the 2004 National Institutes of Health Conference identified six fundamental elements of celiac disease management (referred to by the mnemonic CELIAC): consultation with a skilled dietician, education about the disease, lifelong adherence to a gluten-free diet, identification and treatment of nutritional deficiencies, access to an advocacy group, and continuous long-term follow-up by a multidisciplinary team.[5,8] Primary treatment goals include relieving symptoms, healing the intestine, and reversing the consequences of malabsorption, while enabling the patient to follow a healthy, interesting, and practical gluten-free diet.[8,11] Patients usually experience clinical improvement within days or weeks of gluten-free observance.[1]

Patients with celiac disease must adhere to a life-long gluten-free diet (i.e., avoid wheat, barley, rye and perhaps oats) and avoid ingesting gluten from other sources. It is important to remind patients and healthcare providers that maintaining a gluten-free diet means not

### Table 12.3. Examples of Gluten-Free Grains and Flours [8,15]

| | | |
|---|---|---|
| Amaranth | Millet | Sorghum |
| Buckwheat | Potato flour | Soybeans |
| Corn | Quinoa | Teff |
| Flax | Rice | Tapioca |

ingesting foods or any other substances that contain, have been contaminated with, or have come in contact with gluten. Recent reports reveal that it appears that 50 mg of gluten/day is the minimum dose required to produce measurable damage to the small intestinal mucosa in patients with celiac disease.[12] Some clinicians have suggested that the ingestion of even smaller doses of gluten may be problematic. Fortunately, patients can obtain a number of gluten-free grains and foods, and more gluten-free foods are becoming available[8] (Table 12.3).

The intestinal lesions found in patients with celiac disease (characterized by architectural and inflammatory changes of the mucosa of the proximal small intestine) may reduce absorption capacity, placing celiac disease patients at risk for the development of malabsorptive syndrome (including steatorrhea, weight loss or failure to thrive, bloating, flatulence, multiple deficiency states, etc.). Therefore, patients should be assessed for deficiencies of vitamins and minerals. It is particularly noteworthy that deficiencies of folic acid, vitamin B12, fat soluble vitamins, iron, and calcium be considered.[1] Clinicians have reported that iron-deficiency anemia may be the patient's only manifestation of celiac disease in the absence of diarrhea.[13] Unfortunately, the majority of adults with celiac disease have some degree of bone loss resulting in osteopenia or osteoporosis; therefore, it is recommended that all celiac disease patients be screened for bone loss.[3]

Additional study is needed to determine the degree of impact that celiac disease related intestinal damage may have on the systemic absorption of orally administered drugs. It seems reasonable to assume that the absorption of drugs that are absorbed from the proximal portion of the small intestine may be affected by celiac disease-related damage to this organ. Clinicians may also need to consider if the systemic absorption of orally administered drugs may be adversely influenced by chronic diarrhea that occurs in some patients. The clinical significance of decreased drug absorption secondary to intestinal damage and changes in absorption that may occur as the intestine heals may be worthy of study.

## Gluten and Pharmaceutical Products

Patients with celiac disease and healthcare providers must consider the gluten content of all pharmaceutical products that may be ingested.[14] Because gluten is not absorbed through the skin (although it has been suggested that systemic absorption of topically applied products may occur in patients with dermatitis herpetiformis), products that are intentionally, or may inadvertently, be ingested are of particular interest when considering gluten content.[2] Orally ingested prescription drugs, non-prescription drugs, vitamin and nutritional supplements, and health and beauty aids and cosmetics that may be ingested must all be considered.[15] For example, patients may need to be reminded that some lipstick products contain gluten and that wearing lipstick results in swallowing some lipstick and the ingestion of an overlooked source of gluten.

Confirming that a pharmaceutical product is gluten-free may be challenging. Few prescription and non-prescription drug products are labeled as gluten-free. In addition, the ingredient listing on the label may not enable the healthcare provider or patient to conclude if the product is safe for use by celiac disease. Assessing whether a drug, vitamin, nutritional supplement, or a health and beauty aid is acceptable for use by these patients includes the consideration of the product's inherent gluten content, as well as determining if the product may have been contaminated with, or came in contact with gluten. Pharmacists play a significant role and have an important responsibility to assist patients and their caregivers to determine if gluten-free adherence will be compromised by the use of a specific pharmaceutical product.

Patients (and at times healthcare providers) may not recognize the impact that inactive ingredients that are utilized during the manufacturing of a pharmaceutical product may have upon its gluten content. Inactive ingredients that are obtained from whole grains, grain flour, or starch grain may be sources of gluten. Excipients such as corn or potato starches should be gluten-free (unless contaminated with gluten); however, unspecified starch or pre-gelatinized starch, dusting powder, and flour may be obtained from wheat.[16, 17]

The source of sweeteners used in pharmaceutical products must also be investigated. Uncontaminated sucrose, honey, dextrose, fructose, and corn syrup solids should not be problematic; however, other sweeteners such as barley-based brown rice syrup and wheat-based dextrin and maltodextrin must not be ingested by patients with celiac disease.[17]

Fillers, thickening agents, and polymers used for liquid and solid dosage forms such as gums (e.g., acacia, agar, alginates, carrageenan, gellan gum, guar gum, xanthan gum), cellulose, and its derivatives (e.g., hydroxypropylcellulose, methylcellulose, microcrystalline cellulose, sodium carboxymethycellulose), and other polymers (e.g., polyvinylpyrrolidone, crospovidone, croscarmellose sodium) generally do not contain gluten. The source of the solvent or vehicle (alcohol, polyethylene glycol, propylene glycol, glycerin, etc.) used in liquid dosage forms must also be verified for patients who avoid all products made from gluten-containing grains.[17] As with all other products the potential for gluten contamination must be considered.

Crowe and Falini reported that five percent of pharmaceutical companies that responded to a survey published in 2001 stated that they have a policy of producing gluten-free products. The researchers also noted that many pharmaceutical companies who responded to their survey believed that their products were gluten-free, but these same firms did not state that they could confirm that assumption. Some respondents who did not confirm that their products were gluten-free did state that they add no ingredients derived from wheat, rye, barley, spelt, or oats. A number of the manufacturers reported that they could not confirm that their finished products did not contain gluten because the suppliers of the raw materials used in manufacturing the dosage form were not able to guarantee that the materials that they provided were free of gluten. Some of the pharmaceutical manufacturers also stated that they used potato or corn-based starch derivatives in their products, but they were not absolutely sure if minute amounts of gluten contaminants from other raw materials used at the same locations were present in their inactive ingredients.[16] A newer updated survey of the pharmaceutical industry would hopefully reveal that more confirmed gluten-free pharmaceuticals are being manufactured today than at the time of this study.

Patients with celiac disease must also be advised to be cautious when taking non-prescription drugs, vitamins, and minerals. Carefully reading the labels of these products may not confirm whether the product is gluten-free. Dietary supplements must also be discussed with the patient because these products may be promoted as a means of providing a therapeutic benefit; however, they are not drugs and therefore are not regulated in the same manner that drugs are. Care must be taken to ensure that the use of a particular dietary supplement (teas, protein drinks, tablets, drinks, etc.) is acceptable for the patient and that they are aware that a dietary supplement is not a substitute for eating a nutritious and balanced gluten-free diet.[3] It is also extremely important to remind patients that a product labeled as wheat-free may not be gluten-free.

Patients with celiac disease must also check to determine if the health and beauty aids and cosmetics that they use (that have the potential for ingestion) are gluten-free. Although the possible oral ingestion of some of these products may be anticipated (i.e., toothpaste, lipstick, etc.) the potential means by which some products may be delivered to the mouth may be overlooked. For example, while soaps, shampoos, and topical lotions that contain gluten will not be absorbed through the skin, placing one's hands in the mouth while these products are present on the hands, or introducing these products into the mouth through other means (i.e., swallowing shampoo or soap while showering) may result in the ingestion of gluten.[2,3,18] Although not extensively studied, the amount of gluten ingested from a single exposure to a cosmetic, shampoo, or soap will vary and may be small. It must be emphasized however that the patient must make every effort to avoid any ingestion of gluten as the cumulative effect associated with the ingestion of gluten from varied sources may exceed the threshold for causing intestinal damage. Gluten-containing lotions and creams on the hands of individuals who prepare food for consumption by celiac disease patients must also be considered as a means of introducing gluten into food (i.e., contact).

## Obtaining Information about Gluten Content

References that contain information about the gluten content of foods have become more accessible; however, verifying the gluten content of a pharmaceutical product is often still challenging. Web-based listings (i.e., www.glutenfreedrugs.com, www.celiacmeds.com, www.celiaccentral. com, www.ashp.org/gluten) and other publications are available to assist patients with celiac disease and healthcare providers to ascertain the gluten content of some pharmaceutical products.[19] Some professional organizations and celiac disease foundations are also working together (such as the collaborative efforts of the American Society of Health-System Pharmacists and the National Foundation for Celiac Awareness) to assist patients and healthcare providers obtain needed drug information.

When reviewing information concerning the gluten content of a pharmaceutical product, it must always be noted that the product's formulation may have changed since the list of gluten-free drugs that is being consulted was published, and this change may not be reflected in the product's label. Therefore, it is a good practice to periodically check with the manufacturer to ensure that a product that is listed in an online or print reference as being gluten-free is still gluten-free. Labeling statements such as "new formulation," "new product appearance," or "new manufacturer" on a product that was previously designated to be gluten-free should always prompt the patient and healthcare provider to check with the manufacturer to determine if the product is still gluten-free.[16,19] Providing the drug's lot number is helpful when making an inquiry with the manufacturer.[16] As noted previously, although no gluten may be added to a product and a safe grain-based starch may be used in the formulation of the dosage form, a lack of absolute certainty concerning the gluten content of raw materials or potential gluten contamination risks may lead some manufacturers to qualify the information that they provide about a product with statements such as "to the best of their knowledge" the starch used was gluten-free.[3] Additional research is needed to determine the potential adverse events that are associated with the ingestion of trace amounts of gluten by patients with celiac disease.[12]

# Pharmacy Care Considerations

Pharmacists, who are aware of the signs and symptoms of celiac disease, can refer undiagnosed individuals who are manifesting disease-related symptoms for appropriate diagnostic evaluation. Introducing a trial gluten-free diet before obtaining a confirmed diagnosis is not recommended. Clinicians must recognize that all diagnostic tests for celiac disease should be performed while the patient continues to ingest gluten because introducing a gluten-free diet before concluding the diagnostic evaluation may cause serologic tests and biopsies to normalize.[5, 8]

Patients with celiac disease should be encouraged to consult with pharmacists to obtain needed advice and counsel concerning the gluten-free diet, gluten-free drugs, vitamins and nutritional supplements, as well as other health-related matters. Patients known to have celiac disease should be clearly identified in the pharmacy profile system, and care should be taken to always consider the gluten content of prescription drugs and non-prescription drugs that are intended for the patient prior to dispensing. The patient should not be expected to obtain information about the gluten content of their medications. This is the pharmacist's responsibility, which should be carried out on behalf of, and in collaboration with, the patient.

Pharmacists must consider the impact that the diagnosis of celiac disease may have on the patient's lifestyle, as well as emotional and psychological effects that may be associated with the patient learning that they have this disease.[8] Pharmacists should also be prepared to respond to concerns that the patient's family members may have.[20]

# References

1. Green PHR, Cellier C. Celiac disease. *N Engl J Med* 2007;357(17):1731-43.
2. Korn D. Wheat free, worry free: the art of happy, healthy gluten-free living. Carlsbad, NY: Hay House, Inc., 2002.
3. Green PHR, Jones R. Celiac disease: a hidden epidemic. New York, NY: HarperCollins, 2006.
4. Rampertab SD, Pooran N, Brar P, et al. Trends in the presentation of celiac disease. *Am J Med* 2006;119(4):355.e9-355.e14.
5. National Institutes of Health. NIH Consensus development conference on celiac disease. Available at:http://consensus.nih.gov/2004/2004celiacdisease 118html.htm. Accessed February 26 2006.
6. Sollid LM. Coeliac disease: dissecting a complex inflammatory disorder. *Natl Rev Immunol* 2002;2(9):247-55.
7. Drago S, DiPierro M, Catassi M, et al. Recent developments in the pathogenesis, diagnosis and treatment of celiac disease. *Expert Opin Ther Patents* 2002;12(1):45-51.
8. See J, Murray JA. Gluten-free diet: the medical and nutritional management of celiac disease. *Nutr Clin Pract* 2006;21(1):1-15.
9. Catassi C, Kryszak D, Louis-Jacques O, et al. Detection of celiac disease in primary care: a multicenter case-finding study in North America. *Am J Gastroenterol* 2007;102(7):1454-60.
10. Ferrell RJ, Kelly CP. Diagnosis of celiac sprue. *Am J Gastroenterol* 2001;96(12):3237-46.
11. Hallert C, Grant C, Grehn S et al. Evidence of poor vitamin status in celiac patients on a gluten-free diet for 10 years. *Ailment Pharmacol Ther* 2002;16(7):1333-9.

12. Catassi C, Fabiani E, Iacono G, et al. A prospective, double-blind, placebo-controlled trial to establish a safe gluten threshold for patients with celiac disease. *Am J Clin Nutr* 2007;85:160-6.

13. Rodrigo L. Celiac disease. *World Gastroenterol* 2006;12(41):6585-93.

14. Patel DG, Krogh CME, Thompson WG. Gluten in pills: a hazard for patients with celiac disease. *Can Med Assoc J* 1985;133(2):114-5.

15. Gluten-free drugs for celiac disease patients. *Med Lett Drugs Ther* 2008;50:19-20.

16. Crowe JP, Falini NP. Gluten in pharmaceutical products. *Am J Health-Syst Pharm* 2001;58:396-401.

17. Cacace JL. Formulating for the gluten-sensitive individual. *Int J Pharmaceut Compound* 2005;9(5):357-8.

18. Lowell JP. The gluten-free bible: the thoroughly indispensable guide to negotiating life without wheat. New York, NY: Henry Holt and Company, 2005.

19. Plogsted S. Medications and celiac disease-tips from a pharmacist. *Pract Gastroenterol* 2007;58-64.

20. Sverker A, Ostlund G, Hallert C, et al. Sharing life with a gluten-intolerant person-the perspective of close relatives. *J Hum Nutr Diet* 2007;29(5):412-22.

# Circumcision: Ouch!!

*Rita K. Jew*

## Background and Introduction

Circumcision, the surgical removal of the foreskin of the penis, is one of the oldest and most common surgical procedures performed in the neonatal period. Although it is usually performed for religious and ethnic reasons, there is increasing medical literature that describes the potential medical benefits for circumcision. These include decreased risk of urinary tract infections in infants less than 1 year of age, decreased risk of sexually transmitted diseases, and potential decreased risk of penile cancer .[1-2] However, the absolute reduction of urinary tract infection risk is low and other benefits of circumcision can be realized through proper penile hygiene and practice of low risk behavior. Complications associated with circumcision although rare, include bleeding, infection, phimosis, skin bridges, fistula, meatitis, and glan injury.[1-2] Weighing the risks and benefits, the merit of circumcision in the newborn period remains controversial and highly debated. The American Academy of Pediatrics concluded in its policy statement that although scientific evidence demonstrates potential medical benefits of circumcision in the neonatal period, the data are not sufficient to render a recommendation of routine neonatal circumcision.[2]

Nonetheless, once a decision to perform circumcision in a newborn is made, adequate analgesia should be provided. Historically, the debates surrounded the notion of whether neonates and infants feel pain during a procedure, the importance of pain caused by a short procedure and hence whether analgesia is needed. Considerable evidences are now available demonstrating that circumcision without analgesia would result in pain and physiologic stress in the neonate. Changes in heart rate, blood pressure, oxygen saturation, and cortisol levels are some of the physiological responses that result from circumcision pain.[3-6] The American Academy of Pediatrics recommended that some type of analgesia should be used during circumcision.[2] So what is the analgesic of choice for circumcision?

## Analgesic Options

At one time, sweet wine on gauze sucked by the infant was the analgesia of choice for circumcision during religious ceremony. Today, our options include acetaminophen, eutectic mixture of local anesthetics (EMLA®) cream, liposomal lidocaine 4% (L-M-X™4) cream, sucrose pacifier, and penile nerve block.

## Acetaminophen

In a prospective, randomized, double-blind, placebo-controlled clinical trial that included 44 healthy full-term neonates, 15 mg/kg/dose of acetaminophen or placebo were administered 2 hours before circumcision and every 6 hours for 24 hours after circumcision.[7] Intra-operative heart rate, respiratory rate, and crying time were monitored. Post-operative comfort score and feeding behavior were observed at 30, 60, 90, 120, and 360 minutes and at 24 and 48 hours if the neonates were still hospitalized. Compared to baseline, both the acetaminophen group and the placebo group showed significant increase in heart rate, respiratory rate, and crying during circumcision, and no clinically significant difference were observed between the two groups. Post-operative comfort scores were not significantly different until 6 hours post-operatively, when the acetaminophen group had significantly improved scores. Feeding behavior deteriorated in both breast-fed and bottle-fed neonates in both groups, and acetaminophen had no effect on feeding behavior. The authors concluded that acetaminophen did not ameliorate intra-operative or immediate post-operative pain of circumcision.

## Eutectic Mixture of Local Anesthetics (EMLA®) Cream

EMLA® cream, a eutectic mixture of local anesthetics, contains 2.5% lidocaine and 2.5% prilocaine. It is a topical anesthetic agent used for minor procedures such as intravenous cannulation or venipuncture. For maximal effect, approximately 1-2 g of the cream should be applied to the area of the procedure and the area then wrapped with an occlusive dressing (i.e., Tegaderm) for at least 60 minutes. Potential adverse effects of EMLA® cream include blanching of the area of application, methemoglobinemia, and lidocaine toxicity.[8]

A meta-analysis of three randomized, placebo-controlled trials, conducted by the Cochrane Review best summarized the data on the efficacy of EMLA® cream for circumcision.[9] The meta-analysis, which included 139 neonates, showed that compared to baseline, EMLA® cream resulted in a significantly lower elevation in heart rate during various phases of the procedure. Facial activity scores and crying time were also significantly less compared to those with placebo. One study showed significantly higher oxygen saturation in the EMLA® cream group. There was no difference in blood pressure in one study and no difference in crying features in another. Based on these results, the analysis concluded that EMLA® cream can be recommended for routine use during circumcision. The review also concluded that EMLA® cream is safe for use during circumcision.[9]

Prilocaine in EMLA® cream has been associated with methemoglobinemia.[8,10] Two cases of methemoglobinemia have also been reported after the use of EMLA® cream for neonatal circumcision.[11-12] However, in a study of 10 normal neonates, one gram of EMLA® cream was applied to the foreskin prior to circumcision.[13] Eight hours later, a statistically significant increase in methemoglobin levels were noted with the highest methemoglobin level being 3 g/L. Nonetheless, the methemoglobin levels did not exceed that of the normal in any of the neonates (> 50 g/L is considered toxic). Other clinical studies have demonstrated similar results.[14-15] Toxicity from lidocaine, the other component of EMLA® cream, may lead to arrhythmia and seizures,[8] and lidocaine-induced seizures after neonatal circumcision have been reported.[16-17]

Neonates have very permeable skin, and the foreskin where EMLA® cream is being applied to is highly vascularized. Therefore, systemic absorption and hence toxicity of lidocaine and prilocaine should be considered when using EMLA® cream as a topical anesthetic agent for neonatal circumcision. Although studies have demonstrated minimal absorption of lidocaine and prilocaine[15] and the clinically insignificant increase in methemoglobin levels[14-15] from EMLA® cream when used for circumcision, one must be mindful that EMLA® cream is only proven to be safe in a controlled environment. Prilocaine and lidocaine toxicities demonstrated through case reports reiterated that the safety of EMLA® cream for neonatal circumcision is dependent on proper application technique and dose and duration of application.

## Liposomal Lidocaine 4% Cream (L-M-X™4 Cream)

Liposomal lidocaine 4% (L-M-X™4) cream has shown similar efficacy compared to EMLA® cream when used as a topical anesthetic agent for intravenous cannulation and venipuncture. It has the advantage of faster onset of action, requiring only 30 minutes of application time prior to procedure. It is also void of adverse effects such as blanching and methemoglobinemia because of the lack of prilocaine as a component.[8]

In an open-label study, L-M-X™4 cream, EMLA® cream, or dorsal penile nerve block (DPNB) were randomly assigned to 54 healthy, term males less than 1 week old during circumcision.[18] Physiological parameters including heart rate, respiratory rate, and arterial oxygen saturation measured by pulse oximetry were monitored at baseline, during drug application, circumcision, and recovery. Based on heart rate, there was no difference in analgesic efficacy between treatments groups. Compared to L-M-X™4 and DPNB, the EMLA® cream group showed a higher mean respiratory rate. Data for oxygen saturation were too small for comparison. Adverse effects were limited to local reactions in one patient from the L-M-X™4 group, two from the EMLA® cream group, and none in the DPNB group. The authors concluded that L-M-X™4 cream is an effective analgesic for newborn circumcision.

## Sucrose Pacifier

Sucrose pacifier has demonstrated analgesic effect in neonates during painful procedures such as venipuncture with minimal adverse effects. In a placebo-controlled, blinded clinical trial, 71 neonates were randomized to water, dextrose 50%, or DPNB during circumcision.[19] The percentage of time crying during procedure, percentage of change in heart rate from baseline, percentage of change with oxygen saturation, and modified behavior pain score were observed. No statistically significant difference was found between the dextrose 50% and the water group in all of the observations. The DPNB group showed significantly lower pain-related measurements. It was concluded that dextrose 50% was no different than placebo and less effective than DPNB for alleviation of pain during circumcision. A similar study that included 119 neonates confirmed the same results.[20]

Eighty healthy, term newborn male infants scheduled for routine neonatal circumcision were enrolled in a prospective, randomized, double-blind, placebo-controlled trial.[21] All infants received DPNB in a circumcision chair with a pacifier. The infants were randomized to four groups. Group 1: new padded circumcision chair, which allowed free movement of extremities without compromising surgical field and is adjustable to infant size, standard DPNB, and pacifier dipped in water; Group 2: rigid plastic circumcision chair, buffered lidocaine for DPNB, and pacifier dipped in water; Group 3: rigid plastic circumcision chair, standard DPNB, pacifier dipped in 24% sucrose solution; Group 4: control group in rigid plastic circumcision chair, standard DPNB, and pacifier dipped in water. Behavioral distress scale (neutral, minimal fuss, moderate fuss, sustained cry) were recorded at baseline, 2 minutes before the injection of lidocaine for the DPNB, during injection of lidocaine, 2 minutes post-injection, 4 minutes post-injection, and during circumcision. Plasma cortisol levels were measured 30 minutes after circumcision. The groups in the new circumcision chair and pacifier dipped in 24% sucrose solution have significantly better behavioral scores during circumcision, but no difference in cortisol levels were detected among neonates of all groups.

Fifty-seven full-term neonates undergoing circumcision were randomized to one of four groups: Mogan procedure with 24% sucrose-dipped pacifier; Mogan procedure with water-dipped pacifier; Gomco procedure with 24% sucrose-dipped pacifier; and Gomco procedure with water-dipped pacifier.[22] EMLA® cream was applied to the penis 1-3 hours prior to cir-cumcision in all infants. Crying and facial grimacing were recorded continuously during the circumcision. The Gomco procedure took two times longer, and more crying and grimacing were noted. Less crying and grimacing were also noted in the 24% sucrose groups compared to the water groups. Based on these results, EMLA® cream with 24% sucrose dipped pacifier should be used before, during, and after circumcision.

Eighty healthy neonates were randomized to one of the four groups: water-dipped pacifier (control); 24% sucrose-dipped pacifier; EMLA® cream or 24% sucrose-dipped pacifier, and EMLA® cream during circumcision.[23] Heart rate, oxygen saturation, and blood pressure were physiologic parameters measured. Behavioral parameters included duration of cry. Physiologic and behavioral parameters showed significant decrease in pain response in all treatment groups compared to the control group. There was less reduction in oxygen saturation in the 24% sucrose group and 24% sucrose with EMLA® cream group. The EMLA® cream group and 24% sucrose with EMLA® cream group also has the lowest mean systolic blood pressure and significantly less crying. No difference in heart rate was noted among all groups. The 24% sucrose-dipped pacifier with EMLA® cream is most effective in reducing pain during circumcision.

## Penile Nerve Block and Ring Block

Dorsal penile nerve block (DPNB) is the most common type of nerve block performed during circumcision. Subcutaneous ring block, the circumferential local infiltration of lidocaine at the midshaft of the penis, is another local anesthesia technique used for circumcision. Sodium bicar-bonate-buffered and non-buffered lidocaine, bupivacaine, and ropivacaine have all been used as local anesthetic agents for penile nerve block and subcutaneous ring block during circumcision, with lidocaine being the most common anesthetic agent used. Conflicting data exist regarding the difference in efficacy of sodium bicarbonate-buffered lidocaine and non-buffered lidocaine for penile nerve block and subcutaneous ring block. It is important to note that lidocaine in combination with epinephrine should never be used for penile nerve block and subcutaneous ring block because epinephrine can cause vasoconstriction, which can in turn lead to necrosis of the penis.[24]

In a prospective, blinded, controlled trial including 50 neonates, ≥34.5 weeks post-menstrual age undergoing circumcision, patients were randomized to DPNB where lidocaine 1% 0.7-1 mL was administered subcutaneously 3 minutes before circumcision or EMLA® cream 0.5 g was topically administered 1 hour prior to circumcision.[25] The primary outcome measure is the neonatal infant pain scale (NIPS) scores, a measurement of five behaviors: facial expression, crying, breathing patterns, arm movement, and state of arousal. Secondary outcome consisted of heart rate and respiratory rate changes. NIPS scores and increase in heart rate from baseline were significantly lower in the DPNB group. There was no apparent difference in the respiratory rates between groups. Adverse effects include erythema in the EMLA® cream group and small hematoma and penile edema in the DPNB group. Neonates who received EMLA® cream demonstrated a greater pain response during circumcision than those with DPNB.

Sixty-two term neonates were randomized in a double-blind study to lidocaine DPNB and placebo cream or EMLA® cream and sodium chloride solution DPNB.[26] Physiologic measures of pain, heart rate and respiratory rate were recorded every 60 seconds during the procedure. Behavioral distress scores were assigned every 30 seconds during the procedure. Respiratory rate was higher in the EMLA® cream group but, the difference was not statistically significant. Distress scores and heart rates were significantly lower in the DPNB group. DPNB appeared to be more efficacious than EMLA® cream in providing analgesia during circumcision.

In a randomized controlled trial comparing subcutaneous ring block, DPNB, EMLA® cream, and placebo during neonatal circumcision, 52 healthy, full-term, male newborns were included.[27] Heart rate and cry were monitored at baseline, drug application, preparation, circumcision, and post circumcision while methemoglobin level was measured 6 hours after surgery. The three treatment groups all had significantly less crying and lower heart rates compared to the placebo group, which demonstrated sustained elevation of heart rate and high-pitched cry during and post-circumcision. Subcutaneous ring block was effective through all stages of the circumcision, whereas DPNB and EMLA® cream were not effective during foreskin separation and incision. Methemoglobin levels were highest in the EMLA® cream group but not clinically significant. The most effective anesthetic is the subcutaneous ring block, with EMLA® cream the least effective but superior to placebo.

## Conclusion

Based on the literature reviewed, acetaminophen is not an effective analgesic agent during or post-circumcision and hence should not be recommended. Subcutaneous ring block appeared to be more effective than DPNB, which in turn is more effective than EMLA® cream or L-M-X™4 cream, which is more effective than 24% sucrose-dipped pacifier alone. The combination of DPNB with 24% sucrose-dipped pacifier during injection of lidocaine and during the procedure seemed to be the most effective analgesic regimen for use during circumcision. EMLA® cream or L-M-X™4 cream with 24% sucrose-dipped pacifier is an appropriate second choice regimen. When determining the analgesia of choice for circumcision, the environment in which the circumcision is performed should be considered. In a busy and less controlled environment, DPNB with 24% sucrose-dipped pacifier may be the better option to avoid toxicity of EMLA® or L-M-X™4 cream due to overexposure. In addition, the onset of action of the local anesthesia is almost immediate, and hence, no wait time is required prior to the procedure. In a controlled environment and when the procedure is performed within 30-60 minutes, EMLA® or L-M-X™4 cream and 24% sucrose-dipped pacifier can be considered. L-M-X™4 cream may be preferred over EMLA® cream due to its faster onset of action and is devoid of the concerns of methemoglobinemia because of the lack of prilocaine in its formulation.

# References

1. Lerman SE, Liao JC. Neonatal circumcision. *Pediatr Clin North Am* 2001;48(6):1539-57.
2. Anonymous. Circumcision Policy Statement. American Academy of Pediatrics. Task Force on Circumcision. *Pediatrics* 1999; 103(3):686-693.
3. Williamson PS, Williamson ML. Physiologic stress reduction by a local anesthetic during newborn circumcision. *Pediatrics* 1983;71:36-40.
4. Gunnar MR, Fischer RO, Korsvik S, et al. The effects of circumcision on serum cortisol and behavior. *Psychoneuroendocrinology* 1981;6:269-275.
5. Rawlings DL, Miller PA, Engel RR. The effect of circumcision on transcutaneous $PO_2$ in term infants. *Am J Dis Child* 1980;134:676-678.
6. Talbert LM, Krayill EN, Potter HD. Adrenal cortical response to circumcision in the neonate. *Obstet Gynecol* 1976;48:208-210.
7. Howard CR, Weitzman ML, Howard FM. Acetaminophen analgesia in neonatal circumcision: the effect on pain. *Pediatrics* 1994;93:641-646.
8. Taketomo CK, Hodding JH, Kraus DM. *Pediatric Dosage Handbook.* 14th ed. Hudson, OH: LexiComp Inc; 2007-2008.
9. Taddio A, Ohlsson K, Ohlsson A. Lidocaine-prilocaine cream for analgesia during circumcision in newborn boys. *Cochrane Database of Systematic Reviews 2000;(2):CD000496.*
10. Tse S, Barrington K, Byrne P. Methemoglobinemia associated with prilocaine use in neonatal circumcision. *Am J Perinatol* 1995;12(5):331-2.
11. Couper RT. Methaemoglobinaemia secondary to topical lignocaine/prilocaine in a circumcised neonate. *J Paediatr Child Health* 2000;36(4):406-7.
12. Kumar AR, Dunn N, Naqvi M. Methemoglobinemia associated with a prilocaine-lidocaine cream. *Clin Pediatr* 1997;36(4):239-40.
13. Law RM, Halpern S, Martins RF, et al. Measurement of methemoglobin after EMLA analgesia for newborn circumcision. *Biol Neonate* 1996;70(4):213-7.
14. Lander J, Brady-Fryer B, Metcalfe JB, et al. Comparison of ring block, dorsal penile nerve block, and topical anesthesia for neonatal circumcision: a randomized controlled trial. *JAMA* 1997;278(24):2157-2162.
15. Taddio A, Stevens B, Craig K, et al. Efficacy and safety of lidocaine-prilocaine cream for pain during circumcision. *N Engl J Med* 1997;336(17):1197-1201.
16. Rezvani M, Finkelstein Y, Verjee Z et al. Generalized seizures following topical lidocaine administration during circumcision: establishing causation. *Paediatr Drugs* 2007;9(2):125-127.
17. Moran LR, Hossain T, Insoft RM. Neonatal seizures following lidocaine administration for elective circumcision. *J Perinatol* 2004;24:395-396.
18. Lehr VT, Cepeda E, Frattarelli DA et al. Lidocaine 4% cream compared with lidocaine 2.5% and prilocaine 2.5% or dorsal penile block for circumcision. *Am J Perinatol* 2005;22(5):231-7.
19. Kass FC, Holman JR. Oral glucose solution for analgesia in infant circumcision. *J Fam Pract* 2001;50(9):785-788.
20. Herschel M, Khoshnood B, Ellman C, et al. Neonatal circumcision: randomized trial of a sucrose pacifier for pain control. *Arch Pediatr Adolesc Med* 1998;152;279-284.

21. Stang HJ, Snellman LW, Condon LM. Beyond dorsal penile nerve block: a more humane circumcision. *Pediatrics* 1997;100(2)e3:1-6.

22. Kaufman, GE, Cimo S, Miller LW, et al. An evaluation of the effects of sucrose on neonatal pain with 2 commonly used circumcision methods. *Am J Obstet Gynecol* 2002;186(3):564-568.

23. Mohan CG, Risucci DA, Casimir M, et al. Comparison of analgesics in ameliorating the pain of circumcision. *J Perinatol* 1998;18(1):13-19.

24. Litman RS. Anesthesia and analgesia for newborn circumcision. *Obstet Gynecol Surv* 2001;56(2):114-117.

25. Butler-O'Hara M, LeMoine C, Guillet R. Analgesia for neonatal circumcision: a randomized controlled trial of EMLA cream versus dorsal penile nerve block. *Pediatrics* 1998;101(4)e5:1-5.

26. Howard CR, Howard FM, Fortune K, et al. A randomized, controlled trial of a eutectic mixture of local anesthetic cream (lidocaine and prilocaine) versus penile nerve block for pain relief during circumcision. *Am J Obstet Gynecol* 1999;18(6):1506-1511.

27. Lander J, Brady-Fryer B, Metcalf JB et al. Comparison of ring block, dorsal penile nerve block, and topical anesthesia for neonatal circumcision: a randomized controlled trial. *JAMA* 1997;278(24):2157-2162.

# 14

# Friend or Foe? Ibuprofen for Patent Ductus Arteriosus

*Allison Jun*

## Background and Introduction

Premature neonates (gestational age less than 40 weeks) are faced with the possibility of a variety of diseases and complications as a result of immature organ development and poor defense mechanisms. Although advances in neonatology have reduced the severity of these diseases, certain conditions still have the potential to be life-threatening. The condition known as patent ductus arteriosus (PDA) refers to the presence of a shunt between the pulmonary artery and the descending aorta. This is intended to be a temporary shunt used during fetal development to bypass the immature lungs, which are unable to oxygenate the fetal blood supply. In a term neonate, soon after birth, the shunt closes in response to an increase in partial pressure of oxygen that occurs with the infant's first breath. The vasculature of the premature neonate is not as sensitive to this change in partial pressure. As a result, the shunt may remain open after birth and is termed a *patent ductus arteriosus*. Symptoms of a PDA can vary in severity and result from the pulmonary over-circulation that occurs as a result of the shunt. Clinically significant PDA results in respiratory distress, metabolic acidosis, bounding pulses, and the presence of a systolic heart murmur.[1,2] As these symptoms can become life-threatening, particularly in a premature neonate, the need for effective treatment is great. When treatment is indicated, there are a few approaches available.

## Treatment Options

When PDA becomes symptomatic, the goal is to reduce pulmonary over-circulation and close the PDA. Fluid restriction is usually the first approach and is accomplished with strict fluid management and the careful use of diuretics. In addition to fluid restriction, respiratory distress is managed via ventilator support and acid-base management. Closing the PDA can be accomplished using two methods. PDA ligation involves creating a physical closure via a surgical procedure. Pharmacologic therapy involves the use of non-steroidal anti-inflammatory drugs (NSAIDs) to close the PDA.[1] Indomethacin and, more recently, ibuprofen lysine are the two NSAIDs approved for this unique indication (Table 14.1). Although indomethacin has been used for years and has well-established data for efficacy and toxicity, ibuprofen lysine is a recent addition to the PDA arsenal. Ibuprofen lysine is FDA-approved for the closure of clinically significant PDA in premature neonates who weigh between 500 and 1500 g and are no more than 32 weeks gestational age when usual medical management has been ineffective.[2]

**Table 14.1. Characteristics of Medications Used to Close Clinically Significant PDA[3]**

|  | Indomethacin | Ibuprofen |
|---|---|---|
| Dose | Day 1: 0.2 mg/kg<br>Day 2-3: 0.1 – 0.25 mg/kg<br>depending on post<br>natal age | Day 1: 10 mg/kg<br>Day 2-3: 5 mg/kg |
| Frequency | 12 – 24 hr | 24 hr |
| Half – Life | 20 hr | 24 – 48 hr |
| Administration | IV over 20 – 30 min | IV over 15 min |
| Monitoring | BUN, Scr, UOP, CBC, cardiac<br>function, GI function | BUN, Scr, UOP, CBC, cardiac<br>function, GI function |

Ibuprofen lysine is the injectable form of ibuprofen. L-lysine is used to create a water-soluble salt suitable for intravenous administration.

NSAIDs exert their action at the ductus by causing the vasculature to constrict. It is thought that the inhibition of the enzyme, cyclooxygenase, results in a reduction in formation of prostacyclines and prostaglandins, such as prostaglandin E2 (PGE2). PGE2 is a potent vasodilator and is responsible for keeping the ductus open during fetal life.[1,2,3] For years, indomethacin was the only pharmacologic option available for treatment of PDA. Its efficacy has been well established over the years. However, in addition to its therapeutic effect, indomethacin has the potential for toxicity as well. Mainly, it has the propensity to cause significant renal dysfunction. Because a premature neonate is already born with compromised renal function due to organ immaturity, this side effect is undesirable and can result in long-term renal impairment and can predispose the neonate to potential toxicity of renally excreted medications. In addition, indomethacin has been associated with adverse effects on the gastrointestinal tract of the neonate.[3] Bowel perforation is a very dangerous complication of indomethacin therapy, and premature neonates are already susceptible to gastrointestinal complications of prematurity, such as necrotizing enterocolitis. The side effect profile of indomethacin is especially undesirable in this little population.

When ibuprofen lysine was approved for the treatment of clinically significant PDA, it offered another pharmacologic option. It is marketed as a less toxic alternative to indomethacin because it resulted in less renal dysfunction in comparative clinical trials.[2] Table 14.2 provides a summary of the comparative trials between indomethacin and ibuprofen for PDA. The literature indicates that ibuprofen lysine and indomethacin have equivalent efficacy.[4,5,6] In comparative trials, they had a ductus closure rate of approximately 60–70%. In a Cochrane meta-analysis,

## Table 14.2. Clinical Studies Comparing Ibuprofen to Indomethacin for Treatment of Clinically Significant PDA[4,5,6]

| | Van Overmeire | Lago | Su |
|---|---|---|---|
| Objective | Compare ibuprofen to indomethacin for safety and efficacy in preterm infants with PDA | Compare efficacy and safety of ibuprofen and indomethacin for PDA closure | Compare efficacy and safety of ibuprofen and indomethacin for PDA closure in extremely premature neonates |
| Study Design | Randomized controlled trial<br><br>N = 148<br><br>Gestational Age 24 – 32 weeks<br><br>Echocardiograph- confirmed PDA<br><br>Respiratory distress syndrome | Randomized controlled trial<br><br>N = 175<br><br>Gestation ≤ 34 weeks<br><br>Echocardiograph-confirmed PDA<br><br>Respiratory distress syndrome | Randomized controlled trial<br><br>N = 119<br><br>Gestation ≤ 28 weeks<br><br>Echocardiograph-confirmed PDA<br><br>Respiratory distress syndrome<br><br>Treatment to begin within first 24 hours of life |
| Treatment Course | Indomethacin 0.2 mg/kg q 12 hr x 3 doses<br><br>Ibuprofen 10 mg/kg x 1 dose then 5 mg/kg x 2 doses at 24 hour intervals | Indomethacin 0.2 mg/kg q 12 hr x 3 doses<br><br>Ibuprofen 10 mg/kg x 1 dose then 5 mg/kg x 2 doses at 24-hr intervals | Indomethacin 0.2 mg/kg x 1 dose, then 0.1 mg/kg x 2 doses at 24-hr intervals<br><br>Ibuprofen 10 mg/kg x 1 dose, then 5 mg/kg x 2 doses at 24 hour intervals |
| Efficacy | PDA Closure: Indomethacin 66% Ibuprofen 70% | PDA Closure: Indomethacin 69% Ibuprofen 73% | PDA Closure: Indomethacin 88.3%, Ibuprofen 88.1%<br><br>Reopening of ductus after first course: Indomethacin 13.6%, Ibuprofen 15%<br><br>Requirement for surgical ligation: Indomethacin 8.5%, Ibuprofen 6.7% |
| Safety | Oliguria: Indomethacin, 14 patients Ibuprofen, 5 patients | Oliguria: Indomethacin 15%, Ibuprofen 1% | Oliguria: Indomethacin 15.3%, Ibuprofen 6.7% |
| Conclusions | Ibuprofen as efficacious as indomethacin for PDA closure<br><br>Ibuprofen resulted in less renal dysfunction compared to indomethacin | Ibuprofen as effective as indomethacin for PDA closure.<br><br>Ibuprofen less likely to cause renal dysfunction | Ibuprofen and Indomethacin equally efficacious.<br><br>No significant difference in renal dysfunction or other premature complications |

it was also determined that the two drugs have similar success rates in regard to ductus closure.[1] With regard to renal function, the clinical trials did show a trend of less oliguria; however, this trend was not always statistically significant. Additionally, the trials did not show a difference in gastrointestinal adverse effects between indomethacin and ibuprofen.[4,5,6]

# Children's Hospital of Orange County

Children's Hospital of Orange County (CHOC) is a regional health system, which includes a state-of-the-art 232 bed main hospital facility in the city of Orange, California. The hospital provides services in all areas of pediatrics including medicine, surgery, intensive care, cardio-vascular intensive care, oncology, and neonatal intensive care. Our neonatal intensive care unit (NICU) is a 42-bed unit that provides many levels of care ranging from extracorporeal membrane oxygenation (ECMO) and surgery to home transition care. Newborns that need critical tertiary and quaternary care — most often premature babies suffering from respiratory and circulatory problems — can be admitted just minutes after birth.

After it received FDA approval and was available for use, our institution's neonatal intensive care unit decided to use ibuprofen lysine as the first line pharmacologic treatment for clinically significant PDA. Due to a sudden and well-timed price increase of indomethacin, which is marketed by the same company as ibuprofen, the costs of the two agents were comparable. Since October 2006, we have collected data on all patients who received the drug at our institution. During that time, we used ibuprofen lysine to treat PDA in 30 neonates. As outlined in Table 14.3, the neonates' gestational ages ranged from 23 weeks to 34 weeks. The efficacy rate was similar to that reported in clinical studies. While the remainder of those patients treated ultimately required surgical ligation, the majority of surgical patients had a gestational age of less than 28 weeks. Because this patient population is extremely premature, it is not surprising that the ductus is more resistant to pharmacologically induced closure. This was also observed at our institution in the past with indomethacin-treated patients.

With regards to toxicity of ibuprofen in our patient population, we did not observe an overall significant increase in renal adverse effects. Although 17% of patients treated developed renal failure at some point after ibuprofen therapy, it is important to note that this observation

**Table 14.3. Children's Hospital of Orange County (CHOC) Experience with Ibuprofen for Clinically Significant PDA**

| | |
|---|---|
| Number of Patients Treated | 30 Patients |
| Gestational Age Range | 23– 34 weeks |
| PDA Closure Achieved | 63% |
| Renal Failure | 17% |
| Average Change in Scr | +0.2 mg/dL |
| Average Change in UOP | +0.26 mL/kg/hr |

was not directly linked to ibuprofen use and could be due to several factors. Those patients who developed renal failure may have had other predisposing risk factors. Overall, there was not a significant change in serum creatinine or urine output up to 48 hours after the last dose was administered, indicating that ibuprofen did not have a negative effect on renal function. Also of concern, gastrointestinal adverse effects were monitored closely. We did not notice an alarming number of gastrointestinal adverse effects and were extremely cautious about using it in patients who appeared to be exhibiting early signs of necrotizing enterocolitis.

## Unanswered Questions

As with any new drug, there are some questions that arose after its introduction. In the case of ibuprofen lysine, many questions are still without answers. Often times, after the 3-day treatment course is completed, PDA appears to be smaller than it was, but not completely closed. The symptoms are less severe than they were before treatment, but still exist in a milder form. At this point, the practitioner is faced with making a decision about further treatment. Should we watch and wait? Should we surgically ligate it? Should we start another round of pharmacologic treatment? If so, should we repeat ibuprofen or switch to indomethacin? There are many factors that need to be considered. Is the patient showing any signs of toxicity from the treatment? Is the ductus size unchanged? Are the symptoms of the PDA more severe now than they were when therapy started? There is very little data regarding repeat dosing with ibuprofen. At our institution we have used repeat dosing on one third of our ibuprofen-treated patients. This practice was somewhat inconsistent in that both ibuprofen and indomethacin were used as repeat pharmacologic treatment. Additionally, we needed to educate practitioners on the unnecessary use of another loading dose for the second ibuprofen course if it has been 24 hours or less since the last dose. Anecdotally, it appears that neonates who weigh less than 1000 g often seem to require a repeat course and/or surgical ligation to completely close the ductus. These small patients are at an increased risk for toxicity and exposing them to more intravenous NSAIDs may cause more harm. At this point, the practitioner dictates what to do next. Data is not available to help guide that decision. The risks of a repeat course need to be weighed against the potential benefits. At our institution, if the patient still has PDA but is improving and is not showing signs of toxicity, a repeat course is ordered. If the patient appears to be getting worse or is showing signs of renal dysfunction or gastrointestinal adverse effects, surgical ligation is likely to be the next step.

Another unanswered question is related to an optimal patient population. As mentioned, certain patients are more likely to suffer from toxicity and are therefore not good candidates to receive pharmacologic therapy. An intravenous NSAID is a potent vasoconstrictor and the line between therapy and toxicity can be very fine, especially when administering it to such a fragile patient population. Some may advocate the use of pharmacologic treatment for any patient with PDA. In fact, if an echocardiogram was performed on all neonates soon after birth, the majority of neonates would have a PDA on the first day of life. In most of these cases, the PDA closes on its own during the first 24 hours of life without treatment or evidence of clinical significance. If those patients were to receive empiric treatment with ibuprofen or indomethacin, they would be exposed to the toxicity of these drugs at a vulnerable time. At our institution, the patient is considered for treatment if he or she shows signs of clinically significant PDA. The diagnosis is confirmed with an echocardiogram. After the diagnosis is confirmed, the prescriber then decides if the patient can tolerate the potential toxicity of the drug. Specifically, if the patient is already showing early signs of renal dysfunction (elevated serum creatinine or low urine output) or gastrointestinal distress (abdominal distension or discoloration), he or she will not receive treatment with an intravenous NSAID. As mentioned earlier, the smallest patients tend to be less responsive to pharmacologic therapy. Their vasculature may be more inclined to keep the ductus open. With all of these factors in mind, the optimal patient population may be defined based on gestational age and predisposition for toxicity. This has yet to be determined.

## Intraventricular Hemorrhage Prophylaxis

While it is not the standard of therapy, indomethacin is used by some practitioners to prevent intraventricular hemorrhage (IVH). IVH is another complication of prematurity and results from alterations in cerebral blood flow. There is some evidence to support the use of indomethacin to prevent this complication, and it is occasionally used on the very low birth weight population (less than 1500 g) for this indication.[7] It is hypothesized that the vasoconstrictive effect of indomethacin helps to regulate cerebral blood flow to prevent IVH. Ibuprofen lysine, however, does not seem to share this potential benefit. Available data does not support the use of ibuprofen to prevent IVH, and it is not marketed for this indication. In a study evaluating the effect of intravenous ibuprofen on blood flow to various organs, Pezzati and colleagues demonstrated that cerebral blood flow was not affected by the administration of ibuprofen, indicating that it would not have any protective effect against IVH.[8] Additionally, if the neonate already has a documented or suspected IVH, both ibuprofen and indomethacin are actually contraindicated because they may worsen bleeding complications.[2,3]

### Table 14.4. Contraindications to Ibuprofen Use for PDA[3]

Untreated proven or suspected infection

Congenital heart disease where patency of the PDA is necessary
for pulmonary or systemic blood flow

Bleeding (especially with active intracranial hemorrhage or GI bleed)

Thrombocytopenia

Coagulation defects

Proven or suspected necrotizing enterocolitis (NEC)

Significant renal dysfunction

Hypersensitivity to Ibuprofen or NSAIDs

## Practical Considerations

At our institution, we have educated pharmacy, nursing, and medical staff on the practical use of ibuprofen lysine. The medication has several contraindications that are listed in Table 14.4. In addition, ibuprofen is still an anti-inflammatory medication and can therefore mask the signs and symptoms of infection, which means that healthcare professionals need to be more diligent about evaluating the patient for infection. That being said, the intravenous form of ibuprofen does not carry the indication for treatment of fever or pain. It has not been evaluated for efficacy and safety for that indication. Additionally, the oral form of ibuprofen is not indicated for treatment of clinically significant PDA. The intravenous product is the only form extensively studied and approved for this indication. Another potential complication of therapy may occur as a result of ibuprofen displacing bilirubin from its albumin-binding site.[3] This is a theoretic complication, and we have not seen this result in hyperbilirubinemia at our institution. Another complication that is mentioned more often is the potential for renal dysfunction. While it is marketed as a less toxic agent on the kidneys, it still has the potential to cause renal complications. As such, it is recommended that if the patient becomes anuric or if urine output drops to less than 0.6 mL/kg/hr, ibuprofen therapy should be held until urine output improves.[3]

## Summary

Our NICU was looking forward to using ibuprofen for treatment of clinically significant PDA ever since the drug was approved in Europe and shown to cause less renal dysfunction than indomethacin. When it was approved and available in the United States, we were eager to get experience with it and, hopefully, see better patient outcomes. Due to the relatively low number of patients with whom we have used it, the benefits of ibuprofen over indomethacin are not clear. However, according to the literature and our limited experience, the drug appears to be as efficacious as indomethacin and may cause less toxicity. Practitioners using the drug for this indication should familiarize themselves with its use and contraindications as well as the practical issues related to the drug. Healthcare professionals need to be diligent in identifying patients who may not be optimal candidates for treatment with ibuprofen lysine due to predisposing factors to toxicity. Additionally, because the smallest premature neonates are less likely to respond to one course of pharmacologic therapy, practitioners must weigh the risks versus benefits of repeating the treatment course. As with any new drug, there are many questions that remain unanswered until more experience is gained. As our institution and other institutions gain more experience with ibuprofen lysine, we will continue to analyze the data to answer these questions—with the ultimate goal of providing optimal therapy with little toxicity to each neonatal patient.

## References

1. Ohlsson A, Walia R, Shah S. Ibuprofen for the treatment of patent ductus arteriosus in preterm and/or low birth weight infants. *Cochrane Rev* Jan 9, 2005.
2. Neoprofen package insert and formulary information 5/06

3. Lexi-Comp Online™, Pediatric Lexi-Drugs Online™, Hudson, Ohio: Lexi-Comp, Inc.; 2006; May 30th, 2006

4. Van Overmeire B, Smets K, Lecoutere D, et al. A comparison of ibuprofen and indomethacin for closure of patent ductus arteriosus. *N Engl J Med* 2000;343:674-81.

5. Lago P, Bettio T, Salvadori S, et al. Safety and efficacy of ibuprofen versus indomethacin in preterm infants treated for patent ductus arteriosus: a randomised controlled trial. *Eur J Pediatr* 2002;161:202-207.

6. Su B, Lin H, Chui H, et al. Comparison of ibuprofen and indomethacin for early-targeted treatment of patent ductus arteriosus in extremely premature infants: A randomized controlled trial. *Arch Dis Child Fetal Neonatal Ed* 2007 Sept 3 (E Pub).

7. Ment L, Oh W, Ehrenkranz R, et al. Low-dose indomethacin and prevention of intraventricular hemorrhage: a multicenter randomized trial. *Pediatrics* 1994;93(4):543-50.

8. Pezzati M, Vangi V, Biagiotti R, et al. Effects of indomethacin and ibuprofen on mesenteric and renal blood flow in preterm infants with patent ductus arteriosus. *J Pediatr* 1999;135:733-8.

# Hyporesponse to Erythropoietic Stimulating Agents: Uh-Oh, What Do We Do Now?

*Sarah Tomasello*

## Background of Anemia of Chronic Kidney Disease

### Pathophysiology

Anemia is an expected complication of chronic kidney disease (CKD) as the kidneys produce nearly all of the body's supply of erythropoietin. This hormone is synthesized and released from the kidneys and travels to the bone marrow stimulating the differentiation and proliferation of erythrocytes from the committed erythroid progenitor cells. As CKD progresses from mild to severe and the kidney becomes less able to synthesize erythropoietin, the degree of anemia generally worsens[1,2] (Fig. 15.1). In fact, anemia may be present even in patients with mild CKD[1], and the vast majority of patients with stage 5 CKD are anemic.[3] Although a relative deficiency or lack of EPO is the primary cause of anemia of CKD, patients may have other types of anemia, comorbid diseases, or other factors that can worsen anemia. Possible secondary causes of anemia will be discussed in detail later in this chapter.

### Prevalence of Anemia of Chronic Kidney Disease

Epidemiologic studies estimate that there are currently more than 20 million people with CKD in the United States.[4-5] Of this CKD population, approximately eleven million have mild disease while more than eight million are considered to have moderate to severe CKD. While this entire population is at risk for anemia, the more severe anemia is likely to occur in those patients with more severe dysfunction. Recent data[3] has shown that nearly 70% of patients were anemic by the time they reached stage 5 CKD. It is important to note that although approximately 30% of these patients were receiving an ESA, the average hemoglobin (Hb) concentration was still below the target range (10.2 g/dL).

### Sequelae

The inability to properly oxygenate the body causes widespread effects in the body that range from mild to severe. Generalized fatigue, malaise, shortness of breath, decreased libido, decreased

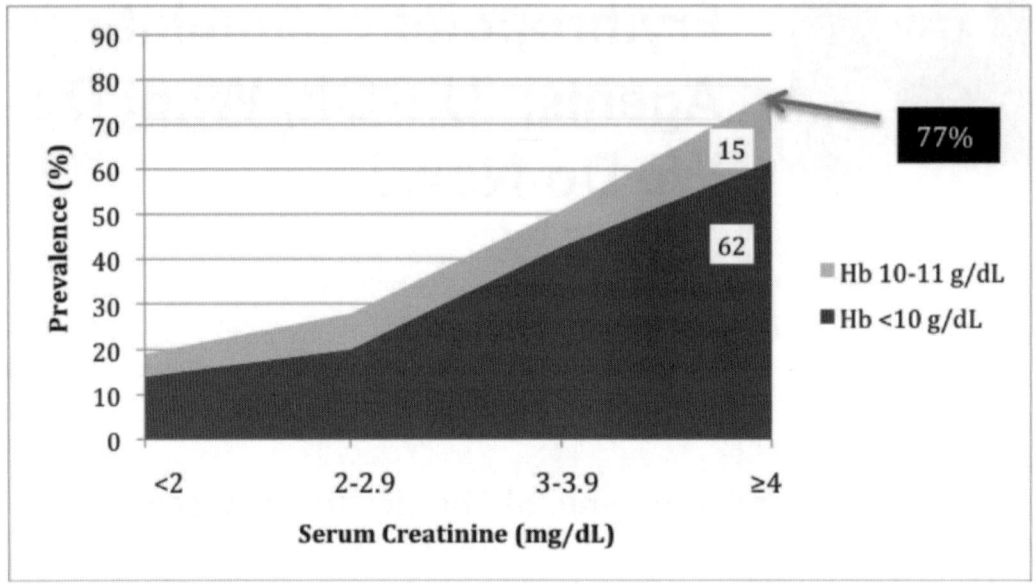

Hb = Hemoglobin

**Figure 15.1.** Relationship of severity of chronic kidney disease to the prevalence of anemia. There is a direct correlation between the severity of chronic kidney disease and the prevalence and severity of anemia. In this study, nearly 20% of patients with a serum creatinine <2.0mg/dL were anemic, while more than 75% of patients with a serum creatinine ≥4mg/dL were anemic. Additionally, the severity of anemia also worsened. When the serum creatinine was <2 mg/dL there were the prevalence of patients with severe anemia (<10mg/dL) was 14%. In contrast, for patients with double that serum creatinine (≥4 mg/dL) the prevalence of severe anemia quadrupled to 62%. Adapted from Kausz AT, Steinberg EP, Nissenson AR, et al. Prevalence and management of anemia among patients with chronic kidney disease in a health maintenance organization. *Dis Man Health Outcomes* 2002:10(8)505-513.

exercise capacity, decreased ability to perform activities of daily living, and decreased quality of life are common symptoms and complaints.[6] The cardiovascular effects of anemia can be even more drastic. To compensate for the diminished oxygen carrying capacity of the blood, there may be an increased chronicity and contractility of the heart. This increased workload may lead to left ventricular hypertrophy (LVH), a risk factor for cardiovascular morbidity and mortality.[7-9] Even in pre dialysis patients with "mild" anemia LVH is prevalent.[7] In a study of 175 patients at a Canadian renal clinic, more than one-fourth of patients with mild CKD had LVH, and 42% of patients with severe CKD had LVH. There is a direct relationship between cardiac function, kidney function, and anemia. As kidney function declines, anemia worsens and hypoxia develops. The heart increases cardiac output to compensate for hypoxia resulting in LVH. Eventually LVH causes a decreased cardiac output and heart failure. The decreased cardiac output leads to decreased perfusion of the kidneys, causing worsening of kidney function and therefore worsening of anemia. The interplay of CKD and heart failure has been coined the "Cardio-Renal Syndrome."[10] In a large epidemiologic study,[11] subjects with CKD and anemia were nearly three times as likely to develop coronary heart disease than those subjects who were not anemic. Additionally, the combination of chronic heart failure, CKD, and anemia increases the risk of death significantly[12-13] (Fig. 15.2).

## Benefits of Treatment

The benefits of treating anemia of CKD may be tremendous. Studies have shown that increasing hemoglobin concentrations can significantly improve subjective quality of life parameters such as assessments of energy, physical function, home management, social activity, and cognitive function.[14-15] Additionally, treating anemia has been shown to slow the progression of CKD,[16] decrease hospitalizations,[17-18] decrease blood transfusions,[18] and decrease healthcare expenditures.[5,19-20] Importantly, treating anemia is associated with regression of LVH[9,11, 21-25] (Fig. 15.3).

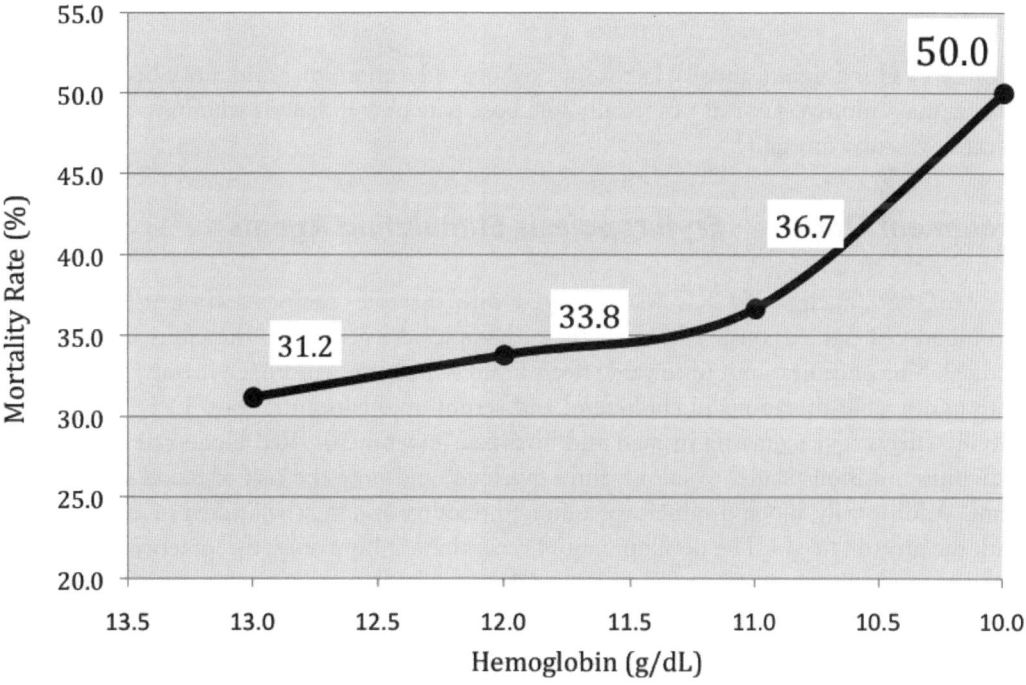

**Figure 15.2.** Mortality rate in patients with both chronic heart failure and anemia. Patients with chronic heart failure and anemia have a significantly increased rate of death. There is a progressive increased risk of mortality as the hemoglobin decreases from 13g/dL down to 11.0g/dL. There is a dramatic increase in the mortality rate in patients with Hb concentrations less than 10g/dL.

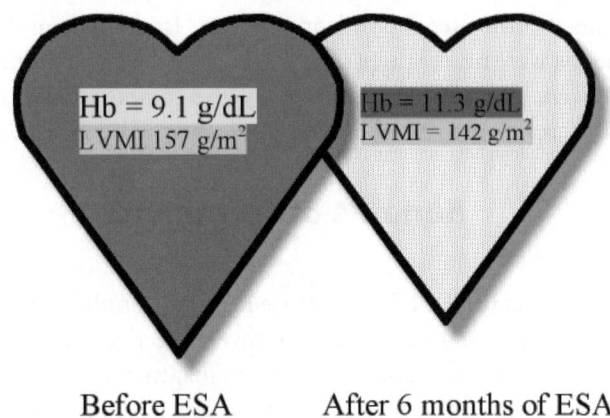

Before ESA          After 6 months of ESA

**Figure 15.3.** In a study of 40 anemic and 61 non-anemic patients, the use of epoetin alfa and increase in hemoglobin was associated with a significant improvement in left ventricular hypertrophy. The left ventricular mass index decreased significantly in the patients with anemia who were treated, versus the control group that were not anemic at baseline. Hb=Hemoglobin, LVMI=Left Ventricular Mass Index.

Because LVH is a significant risk factor for cardiovascular morbidity and mortality, improving anemia may improve survival[16] especially for those patients on dialysis who have a higher risk of cardiovascular mortality.

## Treatment Options – Erythropoiesis Stimulating Agents

Prior to 1989, anemia of CKD was managed with therapies such as androgens and packed red blood cell transfusions. Although these therapies are generally efficacious in increasing hemoglobin concentrations, untoward effects limited their use. Androgen therapy is associated with undesirable alterations in cholesterol and serum lipid concentrations, LVH, and gender specific effects (gynecomastia in men and hirsutism in women). Red blood cell transfusions may cause infusion-related reactions, fluid overload, and pose the risk of blood borne infections. Additionally, blood products are a limited resource and may be limited to those patients with the greatest need. The development of recombinant human erythropoietin in 1989 was a milestone in the treatment of anemia of CKD. Advances in recombinant biotechnology allowed scientists to synthesize erythropoietin using Chinese hamster ovary cells. The first erythropoiesis-stimulating agent (ESA) was marketed in the United States as epoetin alfa.[26] There are two ESAs currently in use in the United States, epoetin alfa (1989) and darbepoetin alfa (2004).[26-27] Both of these agents have been proven to be efficacious in the treatment of anemia in all stages of CKD and are generally well tolerated.[26-27] Unfortunately, although the majority of patients respond to ESA therapy within 2 to 4 weeks and target Hb concentrations may be achieved within a few months,[28-31] approximately 10-20% of patients do not achieve target hemoglobin concentrations.[28,31-32]

The most recent iteration of the National Kidney Foundation-Kidney Disease Quality Outcomes Initiative (K/DOQI™) guidelines regarding the management of anemia were published in 2006.[33] To prepare the guidelines, experts reviewed the available scientific literature regarding anemia of CKD. In addition to providing guidelines and recommendations for the evaluation, management, and monitoring of patients with anemia of CKD, the panel provides a literature review and rationale for each section.

## Treatment Options – Iron Products

Iron is an essential component of hemoglobin; therefore adequate iron delivery to the bone marrow is necessary for optimal erythropoiesis. The KDOQI guidelines[33] recommend evaluating the transferrin saturation percent (or reticulocyte hemoglobin content) and the ferritin concentration as a measure of available iron and stored iron, respectively. Generally the transferrin saturation percent (TSAT) should be maintained between 20-50 and the ferritin concentration should be >100 ng/mL (>200 ng/mL for patients on hemodialysis). Iron deficiency is defined TSAT <20% and/or ferritin <100 ng/mL (<200 for hemodialysis). Unfortunately, the interpretation of these laboratory values, especially ferritin, is complicated.[34] Ferritin is a protein that may bind to iron and act as a storage container by sequestering it in the reticuloendothelial system. Ferritin, however, also acts as an acute phase reactant, and serum concentrations will be elevated in situations of inflammation, infection, or stress. An elevated serum ferritin concentration may therefore indicate an inflammatory process or other condition, not necessarily adequate iron stores. Although there is no clear definition of hyperferritinemia, generally concentrations >500 ng/mL are considered high, and iron products should be used based on the clinical situation with great caution. Functional iron deficiency is the term used to describe the circumstances of a low TSAT (<20%) and an elevated ferritin concentration (>500 ng/mL). A recent study in a hemodialysis population has shown that despite ferritin concentrations between 500-1200 ng/mL, the administration of intravenous iron had beneficial effects on anemia parameters.[35] Intravenous ascorbic acid and L-carnitine are other strategies that have been used to treat functional iron deficiency. These therapies will be discussed in further detail later in this chapter.

The KDOQI guidelines[33] recommend that iron parameters be evaluated routinely in all patients receiving ESA therapy. Iron parameters should be obtained monthly in all patients who have not attained (or maintained) Hb concentrations within the target range. Once the Hb concentration is stable within the target range, iron parameters should be checked at least once every 3 months. Additionally, the guidelines recommend that iron status be evaluated more frequently if based on the clinical situation and professional judgment. More frequent monitoring may be prudent if the patient has received intravenous iron repletion, been hospitalized, had a surgical procedure, or experienced significant blood loss. Additionally, obtaining iron tests may be warranted if the patient requires a significant increase in ESA dose or if the Hb concentration is decreasing despite a constant ESA dose. In fact, iron deficiency (or functional iron deficiency) is a common cause of hyporesponse to ESA therapy. It may be useful to consider iron deficiency as a probable "adverse event" caused by ESA therapy. By enhancing the rate of erythropoiesis, and therefore utilizing more iron, supplementation and repletion of iron will likely be necessary with ESA therapy.

## Definition of Hyporesponse

Unfortunately, not all patients receiving ESAs respond optimally and attain target Hb concentrations. The exact criteria for the diagnosis of *hyporesponse* (or resistance) to ESAs is not well defined in the scientific literature. Generally, it is considered to be a situation in which the hemoglobin concentration is lower than expected for the dose of ESA being given. According to the K/DOQI guidelines[33] regarding the management of anemia, hyporesponse to ESAs should be considered if a significant increase in ESA dose is required to maintain the Hb concentration or, conversely, if the Hb concentration decreases significantly despite a consistent ESA dose. Additionally, hyporesponse should be suspected if the Hb concentration is consistently below the target range despite a sufficient dose of ESA (500 IU/kg/wk of epoetin or equivalent alternative ESA dose). The European Best Practices criteria are slightly more conservative. These guidelines state that resistance to ESAs should be suspected if epoetin doses exceed 300 IU/kg/wk or darbepoetin doses exceed 1.5 µg/kg/wk.[36] Figure 15.4 depicts the recent trend in epoetin dosing from the United States Renal Database.[3]

## Causes of Hyporesponse

There are many factors that can cause or contribute to ESA hyporesponsiveness (Table 15.1). This list of potential causes is extensive, and patients may be affected by numerous factors si-

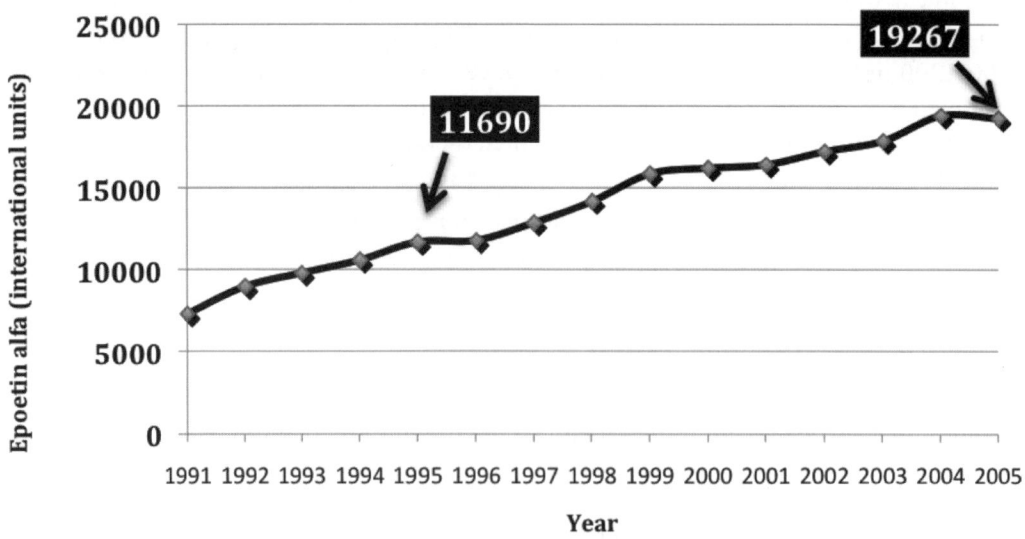

**Figure 15.4.** Trend of increasing weekly epoetin alfa doses in patients with Stage 5 chronic kidney disease. Since 1991 the average weekly epoetin alpha dose has increased steadily in patients with stage 5 chronic kidney disease. In ten years, from 1995 to 2005 the average dose nearly doubled. The increased weekly ESA dose may be a reflection of an increasing incidence of hyporesponse.

multaneously. Identifying the cause(s) can be difficult or impossible. A study of hyporesponsive patients with stage 5 CKD showed that a cause was only identified in 25% of cases.[32] Although some causes may be difficult or impossible to correct (sickle cell disorder, malignancy), many of these secondary causes of anemia are somewhat or completely modifiable (iron deficiency, vitamin deficiency). As noted, a thorough evaluation should be initiated to elucidate all causes of hyporesponse.

## Iron Deficiency and Functional Iron Deficiency

The ESAs act to increase the rate of erythropoiesis. The synthesis of new red blood cells requires iron as an essential part of the heme moiety in hemoglobin. Therefore, it is logical that the iron deficiency may be considered a probable "adverse event" associated with ESA administration. If iron is not supplemented or repleted, erythropoiesis will eventually slow due to deficiency. In fact, patients who are iron replete do not require higher ESA doses.[37]

## Pure Red Cell Aplasia

Pure red cell aplasia (PRCA) is a disorder characterized by the deficiency or complete absence of erythroid progenitor cells in the bone marrow with little or no decrease in other cell precur-

## Table 15.1. Potential Causes of Hyporesponse to ESA Therapy

| | | |
|---|---|---|
| Infection | Autoimmune Disease | Blood loss |
| Acute infection | Systemic Lupus Erythematosus | Surgery |
| Chronic Infection | Rheumatiod arthritis | Gastrointestinal |
| HIV, HepB/C | Vasculitis | bleeding |
| | | Frequent phlebotomy |
| Other Anemias | Vitamin and Mineral Imbalances | Inflammation |
| Sickle cell anemia | **Iron deficiency** | Malignancy |
| Hemolytic anemia | Folic acid | Hypothyroidism |
| Aplastic anemia | Vitamin $B_{12}$ deficiency | Liver disease |
| Pure red cell aplasia | Aluminum toxicity | |
| | Uncontrolled CKD-MBD* | |
| Hemoglobinopathies | Suboptimal dialysis/uremia | Environmental |
| Thalessesmia | | Exposures |
| Sickle cell disease | | Lead |
| Porphyrias | Angiotensin converting | |
| | enzyme-Inhibitors | |
| Anti-cancer agents | Immunosuppressive agents | Hospitalization |

*Uncontrolled chronic kidney disease-related mineral and bone metabolism disorders

sors. This causes a normoblastic, normochromic anemia with a virtual absence of reticulocytes. The disorder may arise from *in utero* stem cell injury (congenital), neoplasm of the thymus gland, or an autoimmune process. The congenital form (Diamond-Blackfan syndrome) is an extreme form of PRCA and is usually accompanied by physical abnormalities and complications. The acquired chronic form is associated with autoimmune diseases such as systemic lupus erythematosus or rheumatoid arthritis. The acute form of PRCA may be drug-induced or triggered by viral infections[6] (Table 15.2). Once triggered, the body produces anti-erythro-poietin antibodies that attack and neutralize ESAs, endogenous erythropoietin and cells with erythropoietin receptors.[33]

The case reports of ESA-induced PRCA that were published in 2002[38] sparked worldwide interest. It was discovered that nearly all of the cases were associated with a preparation of epoetin (Eprex) that was packaged in a syringe with polysorbate 80 and a rubber stopper (not available in the United States). A chemical reaction between the rubber stopper and polysorbate 80 created substances that increased the immunogenicity of the epoetin alfa molecule.[39] The incidence of PRCA spiked from 1998 to 2002, coinciding with the use and cessation of use of the formulation of epoetin described. Although there have not been many reports of PRCA in the United States,[40] pure red cell aplasia remains a concern with the use of epoetin and darbepoetin.[41]

The KDOQI guidelines[33] recommend to assess for pure red cell aplasia if the platelet and white blood cell counts are normal but the absolute reticulocyte count is <10,000 mcL, *and* there is a sudden decline in Hb concentration (0.5 to 1.0 g/dL per week OR the need for regular

### Table 15.2. Potential Causes of Pure Red Cell Aplasia

| Probable causes | Possible Causes |
|---|---|
| Phenytoin | Nonsteroidal anti-inflammatory agents |
| Carbamazepine | Allopurinol |
| Valproic acid | Halothane |
| Azathioprine | Dapsone/pyrimethamine |
| Chloramphenicol | Quinidine |
| Sulfonamides | Gold |
| Isoniazid | Benzene |
| Procainamide | |
| Pesticides | Autoimmune diseases |
| | Chronic lymphocytic leukemia |
| | Chronic active hepatitis |
| | Collagen vascular diseases |

red blood cell transfusions). Additionally, the patient must have been on an ESA for sufficient time to develop antibodies (4 weeks). Pure red cell aplasia causes a sudden, drastic decrease in Hb concentration. Swift recognition and evaluation is imperative as increases in ESA dose will not improve, and may exacerbate, this condition.[26-27]

## Infection/Inflammation

Many circumstances may stimulate the synthesis of endogenous substances that inhibit erythropoiesis. Cytokines are frequently elevated during infections or inflammatory processes, and both have been implicated in the pathogenesis of hyporesponse to ESA therapy.[42-43]

Specifically, tumor necrosis factor alpha, interleukin-1 and interleukin-6, as well as an elevated concentration of C-reactive protein, have been associated with the need for increased dose requirement of ESAs.[44] Hyporesponse has also been correlated with Malnutrition-Inflammation Complex Syndrome. This syndrome is characterized by low total serum cholesterol, pre-albumin, and total iron binding capacity and high concentrations of interleukin-6 and C-reactive protein.[45] Inflammatory cytokines may be stimulated in various situations, such as surgical procedures, vascular access placements and infections,[46-47] and critical illness.[43] Amputations alone have been shown to elicit the inflammatory response and cause hyporesponse to ESAs. Some situations related to infection and inflammation may be modifiable (utilizing arteriovenous fistulas instead of grafts and catheters) while other circumstances are more difficult to improve (eradicating human immunodeficiency virus). Uremia[48] and the hemodialysis HD procedure[49] alone may cause subclinical inflammation. Additionally, administration of intravenous iron compounds may cause oxidative stress and stimulate the inflammatory response.[50]

## Uncontrolled Mineral and Bone Metabolism Disorder

The effects of altered mineral and bone metabolism on anemia management are not completely understood. Alterations in vitamin D, parathyroid hormone, and bone metabolism have all been implicated in the need for higher doses of ESAs.[51-52] Parathyroid hormone may have a direct effect on erythropoiesis by decreasing the production of erythropoietin and/or interfering with the function of the erythroid progenitor cells. Additionally, parathyroid hormone concentrations that are above or below the target range can interfere with normal bone metabolism causing changes in the bone marrow and thereby inhibiting optimal erythropoiesis. There is no direct correlation between serum parathyroid hormone level and ESA dose; however, there is a direct relationship between the severity of bone marrow fibrosis and higher ESA doses.[53] Additionally, and interestingly, a study of hemodialysis patients found that anemia, elevated parathyroid hormone concentrations, and LVH were strongly associated.[54] In cases of severe, refractory hyperparathyroidism, parathyroidectomy has been shown to have a beneficial effect on ESA requirements and Hb response.[55] The role of vitamin D has also not been completely elucidated, but a study has shown that the administration of vitamin D agents can stimulate erythroid progenitor cells and inhibit collagen synthesis to prevent bone marrow fibrosis.[56] Additionally, there may be a correlation between a particular gene polymorphism of the vitamin D receptor (BsmI) and hyporesponse to ESAs. Patients with the BsmI type vitamin D receptor were noted to have a lower Hb and an increased ESA dose requirement than other genotypes.[57]

## Hospitalization

Hospitalization may have a major impact on anemia control of CKD patients.[58] Patients who are acutely ill are likely to have more blood loss, frequent phlebotomy, surgical procedures, vascular access procedures, and gastrointestinal bleeding. Infection, as a cause of hospitalization or acquired during the admission, may be a source of inflammation. Other factors related to worsening of anemia in the hospitalized patient may include length of stay, albumin concentrations, surgical procedures, infections, and frequent phlebotomy. Importantly, the effect of hospitalization may be very significant, and Hb concentrations may remain below target range for several months despite increases in ESA dose.[58]

## Comorbid Diseases

Numerous disease states may cause or worsen anemia. The presence of hemoglobinopathies (i.e., thalassemia, porphyria), malignancies (including chemotherapy and radiation), splenomegaly, chronic liver disease, chronic inflammation (indwelling catheters, amputations), chronic infections (i.e., human-immunodeficiency virus, chronic hepatitis), congestive heart failure, autoimmune diseases (rheumatoid arthritis, systemic lupus erythematosus), malnutrition and vitamin deficiencies, and uncontrolled mineral and bone metabolism disorder are some potential confounders that may complicate the evaluation and treatment of anemia of CKD.

## Drug-Induced Hyporesponse

Many medications can directly or indirectly interfere with optimal erythropoiesis. The most obvious agents are those that cause cell death and damage the bone marrow such as chemotherapeutic agents. Drugs that can decrease the absorption of vitamin $B_{12}$, folate, or iron can cause a secondary anemia to develop.

While some reports suggest that ACE inhibitors negatively effect erythropoiesis,[59] others have not.[60] Both animal and human models have shown that angiotensin II is a potent stimulus for an increased production of erythropoietin.[61-62] In fact, ACE-I may be utilized clinically to treat post-transplant erythrocytosis.[63-64] In one clinical study, patients taking ACE-I had a statistically significant lower Hb concentration than those not taking an ACE-I.[65] Additionally, another study by Naito et al.[66] showed that the decreased erythropoiesis occurs at the level of the erythroid progenitor cell. An *in vitro* study was conducted to compare the effects of an ACE-I to an angiotensin II type I receptor antagonist. The results showed that blockade of the angiotensin II type I receptor caused a greater reduction in erythropoiesis. The use of ACE-I and ARB is prevalent in the CKD population because they are commonly prescribed agents for hypertension and proteinuria. If the use of these agents is a suspected cause of hyporeponsiveness to ESAs, careful assessment of the risk:benefit ratio should be made before discontinuing these agents.

# Evaluation of ESA Hyporesponse

The evaluation of ESA hyporesponse should include all laboratory tests, elements of drug and hospitalization history, and physical examination components necessary to rule out each potential cause of hyporesponse.

# Treatment of ESA Hyporesponse

## *Iron Deficiency – Absolute and Functional*

Absolute iron deficiency is usually easy to diagnose and treat. For patients with decreased TSAT (or CHr) and ferritin concentrations, repletion with iron products is indicated. Administering intravenous iron products in patients with an acute infection, particularly bacteremia, is somewhat controversial due to concerns of worsening infection or supra-infection.[67-69] Additionally, the evidence showing that some intravenous iron products may cause oxidative stress and inflammation must be taken into consideration, and the risk:benefit ratio carefully considered.

While the treatment of absolute iron deficiency is clear, functional iron deficiency is more difficult to assess and manage. As mentioned, serum ferritin concentrations are often interpreted as a marker of iron stores in the reticuloendothelial system. Relying on serum ferritin concentrations can be misleading because ferritin is a serum protein, not necessarily bound to iron, that acts as an acute phase reactant. In situations of inflammation, infection, or other stress, serum ferritin concentrations may be elevated while the movement of stored iron from the reticuloendothelial system to the serum (and bone marrow) is inhibited. Although serum ferritin concentrations may appear elevated (hyperferritinemia), if the transferrin saturation is low there is not sufficient iron readily available for erythropoiesis.

Several strategies have been employed to treat functional iron deficiency. As mentioned, the use of intravenous iron products should be used cautiously in situations of hyperferritinemia (ferritin >500 ng/mL). A recent study has shown that administering a repletion regimen (one gram of sodium ferric gluconate divided into eight doses given on consecutive dialysis days) to patients with hyperferritinemia and Hb less than or equal to 11 g/dL resulted in a statistically significant increase in Hb concentration.[35] Additionally, an extension study followed patients for a total of 12 weeks and found that patient who, received treatment maintained higher Hb concentrations and had fewer adverse events.[70] This trial provides evidence that administering intravenous iron products to patients with functional iron deficiency (TSAT <25% and ferritin up to 1200ng/dL) is effective and safe. While more research is clearly necessary, judicious use of iron may be a valuable tool to manage functional iron deficiency-associated hyporesponse.

## *Pure Red Cell Aplasia*

The treatment and prognosis of PRCA varies. There has been some success using immunosuppressive therapies such as prednisone, cyclophosphamide, or rituximab.[71] Some patients may not be able to resume ESA therapy and may become transfusion-dependent.[72] A long-term follow-up of 170 patients with ESA-induced PRCA showed that of the patients who achieved a hematologic recovery, a higher percentage had received immunosuppressive therapy. This follow-up study also found that the majority of patients who had undetectable levels of antierythropoietin antibodies at the time of subsequent ESA administration did indeed respond to therapy. Fortunately, the incidence of PRCA has declined dramatically since the reformulation of Eprex.[33] Careful attention should be paid, however, to any patient with a dramatic decrease in Hb or increased dose requirement of ESAs.

## Adjuvants to ESA and Iron Therapy

The KDOQI guidelines on the management of anemia of CKD[33] do not recommend the use of any adjuvant therapy due to the lack of evidence of safety and efficacy. The following information is provided for information, knowledge, and research purposes. It is the author's opinion that any of the adjuvants discussed (except androgens) could be used cautiously if other traditional therapy fails and the benefits of adjuvant therapy outweigh the risks.

## Intravenous Ascorbic Acid

Many small studies have explored the efficacy of intravenous ascorbic acid (IVAA) as adjuvant therapy for anemia of CKD in patients on hemodialysis.[73-82] Although the exact mechanism of action is not fully understood, ascorbic acid may alleviate functional iron deficiency by acting as an electron donor to reduce ferric iron (stored) to ferrous iron (available for incorporation into heme moiety) and facilitate movement from the reticuloendothelial system to the serum.[83] The fact that ascorbic acid also acts as an antioxidant is also beneficial given that patients on hemodialysis may have increased markers of inflammation. Clinically, administration of IVAA may result in a decrease in ferritin concentrations and an increase in TSAT. Moving iron from the reticuloendothelial system to the serum provides more iron readily available for erythropoiesis. A subsequent rise in Hb and reduction in ESA dose may be observed.[84]

Generalizing the information gathered from the available studies is complicated. The numbers of patients in the trials were small, the dose of IVAA ranged from 100 to 500 mg given three times a week on hemodialysis, and the duration of therapy ranged from 2 months to 6 months or more. Additionally, the patient population was chosen using different criteria (degree of hyperferritinemia, upper limit of TSAT, Hb concentrations). The definition of efficacy varied in the trials from a significant increase in Hb from baseline to increased quality of life. Perhaps the most difficult barrier to generalizing the results of the available studies is the differences in patient populations. The fact that few studies actually targeted patients with hyporesponse to ESA therapy limits the usefulness of the findings (positive or negative).

Of all of the studies reviewed, two of the studies did not demonstrate any difference in outcomes with the use of ascorbic acid. Chan et. al.[74] compared the intravenous form to the oral form of ascorbic acid with an extension study of oral ascorbic acid versus no treatment. In the first part of the study, 30 patients were selected based on the following parameters: Hb <12g/dL, TSAT <30%, and ferritin concentration >500ng/mL. The patients selected had average baseline Hb concentrations of 11.3 and 11.7 g/dL in the IV and oral groups, respectively. The average baseline epoetin dose was between 148 and 165 U/kg per week. The average ferritin was 658 and 603 ng/mL. The first study (21 patients for analysis) showed no difference between oral and intravenous administration on anemia parameters. Unfortunately, the patients selected would not be classified as hyporesponsive by most of the current definitions.[33,36] The second part of the study was to compare 500 mg of oral ascorbic acid with dialysis to no treatment in 153 randomly chosen hemodialysis patients. Again, interpreting this study is difficult because although the patients were randomized, there was a statistically higher ferritin concentration in the "no treatment" arm, 749 versus 943 ng/mL. As with the first study, the baseline epoetin concentration in both groups was not extreme, 132 and 124 U/kg per week, and the Hb concentrations were approximately 12 g/dL in both arms at baseline and at the end of the study. Although these studies showed little benefit of ascorbic acid for the selected patients, other studies focusing on hyporesponsive patients have shown much benefit. Similar reasoning might explain the findings of a randomized, controlled trial in 61 hemodialysis patients.[78] Thirty patients were randomly selected to receive 100 mg IVAA after hemodialysis for 6 months. Thirty-one patients were randomly selected to act as controls. The primary objective was to assess the difference in quality of life parameters (SF-36) between the groups. Although the SF-36 scores were not statistically different at the completion of the study, the patients were not selected on the basis of hyperferritinemia or hyporesponse to ESA therapy.

The caveat of IVAA use is the risk of oxalosis, the accumulation of oxalate crystals from ascorbate metabolism.[85] The upper limit of serum oxalate concentration of 50 μmol/L has been suggested,[86] however the significance of this has been questioned.[87] There are no reports of clinical adverse events associated with the administration of 100-500 mg of IVAA given at each hemodialysis session for up to 6 months. Intravenous ascorbic acid, however, should not be given to patients with primary or secondary hyperoxaluria.

The KDOQI guidelines of 2006[33] acknowledge the paucity of evidence to support the routine use of IVAA. Based on the fact that there are few studies that targeted hyporesponsive patients with hyperferritinemia, the KDOQI guidelines do not recommend the use of IVAA in the management of anemia of CKD.

## L-Carnitine

L-carnitine plays a number of roles in the body and is essential for proper metabolism and energy production. Carnitine is synthesized from lysine and methionine in the liver, brain, and kidneys.[88] There are two types of carnitine deficiencies. Primary deficiencies are genetically inherited disorders, and patients are generally severely affected. Secondary deficiencies may be caused by inadequate intake (rarely) and synthesis or excessive elimination from the body.[89] Because the body can synthesize carnitine, inadequate consumption of dietary carnitine does not generally cause a deficiency. The balance can be upset, however, in circumstances of increased carnitine excretion. The use of valproic acid and zidovudine has been associated with carnitine deficiency. Of importance, the process of dialysis (both peritoneal and hemodialysis) removes carnitine from the body.

The supplementation of carnitine has been studied for various issues related to CKD and dialysis. Studies have explored the use of carnitine for improving physical function, cardiac disease, hypotension, and anemia. In regard to anemia, it is proposed that carnitine enhances erythrocyte membrane stability and survival.[90] Much evidence from small heterogeneous trials has demonstrated a benefit on anemia parameters. Unfortunately, as with IVAA, the trials are small, and many are non-randomized. Additionally, patients were selected based on variable criteria, and endpoints were not consistent. Although the most recent KDOQI guidelines do not recommend the use of L-carnitine for hyporesponse to ESA therapy, the interested reader is directed to another publication [Am J Kidney Dis 2003; 41(4 suppl 4)] for extensive information regarding its use for various disorders in patients with CKD.

## Pentoxifylline

The exact role that Pentoxifylline plays in improving anemia is not fully elucidated. In addition to acting as a free oxygen radical scavenger.[91] Pentoxifylline has been shown to inhibit the production and action of mediators of inflammation such as tumor necrosis factor alfa and interleukin 6 production.[92] Pentoxifylline has been used to treat anemia of sickle cell disease. In small studies of hemodialysis patients, it has increased hemoglobin concentrations when administered as 400 mg orally every day.[93-94]

## Androgens

Androgens such as fluoxymesterone, testosterone, and nandrolone were frequently prescribed agents to manage anemia of CKD prior to the synthesis of ESAs. Unfortunately, adverse effects such as acne, hirsutism, liver damage and hepatocellular carcinoma, and priapism limited their use. With the availability of ESAs and iron products to manage anemia, the risks outweigh the benefits. The KDOQI guidelines strongly discourage the use of androgens to treat anemia of CKD.[33]

# Conclusion

In conclusion, anemia of CKD may be affected by many factors and concomitant disease states. All contributing circumstances should be identified and corrected/improved if possible. Although not all causes of hyporesponse are curable, easily modifiable causes should be corrected as soon as possible. Careful monitoring, identification, evaluation, and creation of a treatment plan are very important to combating hyporesponse to ESA therapy. A structured team approach has been shown to improve anemia parameters in patients with hyporesponse.[95] Adjuvant therapies may be utilized to maximize response to ESAs and iron therapy.

# References

1. McClellan W, Aronoff SL, Bolton WK, et al. The prevalence of anemia in patients with chronic kidney disease. *Curr Med Res Opin* 2004;20(9):1501-1510.
2. Kausz AT, Steinberg EP, Nissenson AR, et al. Prevalence and management of anemia among patients with chronic kidney disease in a health maintenance organization. *Dis Manage Health Outcomes* 2002;10(8):505-513.
3. United States Renal Data System (USRDS). 2007 Annual Data Report: Atlas of End-Stage Renal Disease in the United States. National Institutes of Health, National Institute of Diabetes and Digestive and Kidney Diseases, Bethesda, MD, 2007.
4. Coresh J, Astor BC, Greene T, et al. Prevalence of chronic kidney disease and decreased kidney function in the adult US population: Third National Health and Nutrition Examination Survey. *Am J Kidney Dis* 2003;41(1):1-12.
5. Collins A, Ebben J, Ma J, et al. Hematocrit levels and associated Medicare expenditures. *Am J Kidney Dis* 2000; 36:282-293.
6. Greer JP, Foerster J, Lukens JN, et al. Eds. Wintrobe's Clinical Hematology, 11th Edition. 2004. Philadelphia, PA; Lippincott Williams and Wilkins, 949-952.
7. Levin A, Singer J, Thompson C, et al. Prevalent left ventricular hypertrophy in the pre-dialysis population: Identifying opportunites for intervention. *Am J Kidney Dis* 1996;27:347-354.

8. Foley R, Parfrey P, Hamett J, et al. The impact of anemia on cardiomyopathy, morbidity and mortality in end-stage renal disease. *Am J Kidney Dis* 1996;28:53-61.

9. Locatelli F. The impact of hematocrit levels and erythropoietin treatment on overall and cardiovascular mortality and morbidity: The experience of the Lombardy Dialysis Registry. *Nephrol Dial Transplant* 1998;13:1642-1644.

10. Silberberg DS, Wexler D, Iaina A. The role of anemia in congestive heart failure and chronic kidney insufficiency: the cardio renal anemia syndrome. *Perspect Biol Med* 2004;47(4):575-589.

11. Silberberg J, Racine N, Barre P, et al. Regression of left ventricular hypertrophy in dialysis patients following correction of anemia with recombinant human erythropoietin. *Can J Cardiol* 1990;6:1-4.

12. Abramson JL, Jurkovitz CT, Vaccarino V, et al. Chronic kidney disease, anemia, and incident stroke in a middle-aged, community-based population: The ARIC Study. *Kidney Intl* 2003;64:610-615.

13. McClellan WM, Flanders WD, Langston RD, et al. Anemia and renal insufficiency are independent risk factors for death among patients with congestive heart failure admitted to community hospitals: a population-based study. *J Am Soc Nephrol* 2002;13(7)1928-1936.

14. Kausz AT, Obrador GT, Pereira BJ. Anemia management in patients with chronic renal insufficiency. *Am J Kidney Dis* 2000; 36(Suppl 3): S39–51.

15. Revicki DA, Brown RE, Feeny DH, et al. Health-related quality of life associated with recombinant human erythropoietin therapy for predialysis chronic renal disease patients. *Am J Kidney Dis* 1995;25:548-554.

16. Jungers P, Choukroun GF, Oualim Z, et al. Beneficial influence of recombinant human erythropoietin therapy on the rate of progression of chronic renal failure in predialysis paitents. *Nephrol Dial Transplant* 2001;16:307-312.

17. Xia H, Ebben J, Ma J, et al. Hematocrit levels and hospitalization risks in hemodialysis patients. *J Am Soc Nephrol* 1999;10:1309-1316.

18. Churchill DN, Muirhead N, Goldstein M, et al. Effect of recombinant erythropoietin on hospitalization of hemodialysis patients. *Clin Nephrol* 1995;43:184-188.

19. Collins A, Li S, St. Peter W, et al. Death, hospitalization, and economic associations among incident hemodialysis patients with hematocrit values of 36 to 39%. *J Am Soc Nephrol* 2001;12:2465-2473.

20. Maddux FW, Shetty S, del Aguila M, et al. Effect of erythropoiesis-stimulating agents on healthcare utilization, costs, and outcomes in chronic kidney disease. *Ann Pharmacother* 2007;41(11):1761-1769.

21. Jones M, Schenkel B, Just J. Epoetin alfa's effect on left ventricular hypertrophy and subsequent mortality. *Intl J Cardiol* 2005;100(2):253-265.

22. Cannella G, La Canna G, Sandrini M, et al. Reversal of left ventricular hypertrophy following recombinant human erythropoietin treatment of anaemic uremic patients. *Nephrol Dial Transplant* 1991;6:31-37.

23. Hampl H, Hennig L, Rosenberger C, et al. Optimized heart failure therapy and complete anemia correction on left-ventricular hypertrophy in nondiabetic and diabetic patients undergoing hemodialysis. *Kidney Blood Pressure Res* 2005;28:353-62.

24. Hampl H, Hennig L, Rosenberger C, et al. Effects of optimized heart failure therapy and anemia correction with epoetin beta on left ventricular mass in hemodialysis patients. *Am J Neprhol* 2005;25(3):211-220.

25. Ayus JC, Go AS, Valderrabano F, et al. Effects of erythropoietin on left ventricular hypertrophy in adults with severe chronic renal failure and hemoglobin <10 g/dL. *Kidney Intl* 2005;68:788-795.

26. Epogen (epoetin alfa) [package insert]. Thousand Oaks. CA: Amgen Inc, 1989-2008.

27. Aranesp (darbepoetin alfa) [package insert]. Thousand Oaks. CA: Amgen Inc, 2008.

28. Abbas EE, Afioni N, Al Wakeel J. The new rHuEPO alpha (epoetin) in the management of anemia of end-stage renal disease in patients on maintenance hemodialysis. *Tranplant Proceed* 2004;36(6) 1805-1811.

29. Nissenson AR, Swan SK, Lindberg JS, et al. Randomized, controlled trial of darbepoetin alfa for the treatment of anemia in hemodialysis patients. *Am J Kidney Dis* 2002;40(1):110-118.

30. Kulzer P, Scheafer RM, Krahn R, et al. Effectiveness and safety of recombinant human erythropoietin (r-HuEPO) in the treatment of anemia of chronic renal failure in non dialysis patients. European Multicentre Study Group. *Intl J Artificial Organs* 1994;17(4):195-202

31. Portoloes J, Lopez-Gomez JM, Aljama, Pedro. Anemia management and treatment response in patients on hemodialysis: the MAR study. *J Nephrol* 2006;19(3):352-360.

32. Kausz AT, Solid C, Pereira B, et al. Intractable anemia among hemodialysis patients: A sign of suboptimal management or a marker of disease? *Am J Kidney Dis* 2005;45(1):136-147.

33. National Kidney Foundation. KDOQI clinical practice guidelines and clinical practice recommendations for anemia of chronic kidney disease. *Am J Kidney Dis* 2006;47(5 suppl 3):s11-s145.

34. Kalantar-Zadeh Ka, Kalantar-Zadeh Ko, Lee GH. The fascinating but deceptive ferritin: to measure it or not to measure it in chronic kidney disease? *Clin J AmSoc Nephrol* 2006;1(suppl 1):s9-18.

35. Coyne DW, Kapoian T, Suki W, et al. Ferric gluconate is highly efficacious in anemic hemodialysis patients with high serum ferritin and low transferrin saturation: results of the Dialysis Patients' Response to IV Iron with Elevated Ferritin (DRIVE) Study. *J Am Soc Nephrol* 2007;18(3)975-984.

36. Locatelli F. Revised European Best Practice Guidelines for the management of anaemia in patients with chronic renal failure. *Nephrol Dial Transplant* 2004;19(suppl 2):sii32-36

37. Pizzarelli F, David S, Sala P, et al. Non-replete hemodialysis patients do not require higher EPO dosages when converting from subcutaneous to intravenous administration: results of the Italian Study on Erythropoietin Converting (ISEC). *Am J Kidney Dis* 2006;47(6):1027-1035.

38. Casadevall N, Nataf J, Viron B, et al. Pure red-cell aplasia and antierythropoietin antibodies in patients treated with recombinant erythropoietin. *N Engl J Med* 2002;346(7):469-475.

39. Boven K, Knight J, Bader F, et al. Epoetin-associated pure red cell aplasia in patients with chronic kidney disease: solving the mystery. *Nephrol Dial Tranplant* 2005;20(suppl 3): iii33-40.

40. Gershon SK, Luksenburg H, Cote TR, et al. Pure red-cell aplasia and recombinant erythropoietin. *N Engl J Med* 2002;346:1584-1585.

41. Jacob A, Sandhu K, Nicholas J, et al. Antibody-mediated pure red cell aplasia in a dialysis patient receiving darbepoetin alfa as the sole erythropoietic agent. *Nephrol Dial Transplant* 2006;21(10):2963-2965.

42. Means Jr. RT. Pathogenesis of the anaemia of chronic disease: a cytokine mediated anaemia. *Stem Cells* 1995;13:32-37.

43. Rogiers P, Zhang H, Leeman M, et al. Erythropoietin response is blunted in critically ill patients. *Intensive Care Med* 1997;23:159-162.

44. Macdougall IC, Cooper A. The inflammatory response and epoetin sensitivity. *Nephrol Dial Transplant* 2002;17(48-52).

45. Kalantar-Zadeh K, McAllister CJ, Lehn RS, et al. Effect of malnutrition-inflammation complex syndrome on EPO hyporesponsiveness in maintenance hemodialysis patients. *Am J Kidney Dis* 2003;42(4):761-773.

46. Roberts TL, Obrador GT, St Peter WL, et al. The relationship among catheter insertions, vascular access infections and anemia management in hemodialysis patients. *Kidney Int* 2004;66(6):2429-2436.

47. Teruel JL, Marcen R, Ocana, Javier, et al. Clinical significance of C-reactive protein in patients on hemodialysis: a longitudinal study. *Nephron* 2005;100(4)140-145.

48. Kaysen GA. The microinflammatory state in uremia: causes and potential consequences. *J Am Soc Nephrol* 2001;12:1549-1557.

49. Borawski J, Pawlak K, Mysliwiec, M. Inflammatory markers and platelet aggregation tests as predictors of hemoglobin and endogenous erythropoietin levels in hemodialysis patients. Nephron 2002;91(4)671-681.

50. Zager RA. Parenteral iron compounds: potent oxidants but mainstays of anemia management in chronic renal disease. *Clin J Am Soc Nephrol* 2006;1(suppl 1):s24-31.

51. Tonelli M, Blake PG, Muirhead N. Predictors of erythropoietin responsiveness in chronic hemodialysis patients. *ASAIO* 2001;47(1)82-85.

52. Neves PL, Trivino J, Casaubon F, et al. Elderly patients on chronic hemodialysis: effect of the secondary hyperparathyroidism on the hemoglobin level. *Intl Urol Nephrol* 2002;34(1):147-149.

53. Al-Hilali N, Al-Humoud H, Ninan M, et al. Does parathyroid hormone affect erythropoietin therapy patients? *Med Principle Pract* 2007;16(1):63-67.

54. Datta S, Abraham G, Mathew M, et al. Correlation of anemia, secondary hyperparathyroidism with left ventricular hypertrophy in chronic kidney disease patients. *J Assoc Physician India* 2006;54:699-703.

55. Lee CT, Chou FF, Chang HW, et al. Effects of parathyroidectomy on iron homeostasis and erythropoiesis in hemodialysis patients with severe hyperparathyroidism. *Blood Purification* 2003;21(6):369-375.

56. Deicher R, Horl WH. Hormonal adjuvants for the treatment of renal anaemia. *Euro J Clin Invest* 2005;35(Suppl 3):75-84.

57. Ertürk S, Kutlay S, Karabulut H, et al. The impact of vitamin D receptor genotype on the management of anemia in hemodialysis patients. *Am J Kidney Dis* 2002;40(4)816-823.

58. Yaqub MS, Leiser J, Molitoris BA. Erythropoietin requirements increase following hospitalization in end-stage renal disease patients. Am J Nephrol 2001;21(5):390-398.

59. Teruel JL, Juarez GF, Marcen R, et al. Effect of Angiotensin-converting enzyme inhibitors on anemia in hemodialyzed patients. *Nephron* 1996;73:113.

60. Piccoli A, Pastori G, Pierobon E, et al. Anti-renin-angiotensin-system drugs and development of anemia in chronic kidney disease. *J Nephrol* 2005;18(5):585-591.

61. Freudenthaler SM, Screeb KH, Körner T, et al. Angiotensin II increases erythropoietin production in healthy human volunteers. *Euro J Clin Invest* 1999;29:816-823.

62. Fisher JW, Samuels AI, Langston JW. Effects of angiotensin and renal artery constriction on erythropoietin production. *J Pharmacol Exp Ther* 1967:157:618-625.

63. Gleiter CH. Posttransplant erythrocytosis: a model for the investigation of the pharmacological control of renal erythropoietin production? *Intl J Clin Pharmacol* 1992;34:489-492.

64. Torregrosa JV, Campistol JM, Montesinos M, et al. Efficacy of captopril on posttransplant erythrocytosis. Long-term follow-up. *Transplantation* 1994;58:311-14.

65. Matsumura M, Nomura H, Koni I, et al. Angiotensin-Converting Enzyme inhibitors are associated with the need for increased recombinant human erythropoietin maintenance doses in hemodialysis patients. *Nephron* 1997;77:164-168.

66. Naito M, Kawashima A, Akiba T, et al. Effects of an angiotensin II receptor antagonist and angiotensin-converting enzyme inhibitors on burst forming units-erythroid in chronic hemodialysis patients. *Am J Nephrol* 2003;23:287-293

67. Sirken G, Raja R, Rizkala AR. Association of different intravenous iron preparations with risk of bacteremia in maintenance hemodialysis patients. *Clin Nephrol* 2006;66(5)348-356.

68. Skaar E, Humayun M, Bae T, et al. Iron-source preference of Staphylococcus aureus infections. *Science* 2004;305:1626-1628.

69. Brewster UC, Coca SG, Reilly RF, et al. Effect of intravenous iron on haemodialysis catheter microbial colonization and blood-borne infection. *Nephrology* 2005;10(2):124-128.

70. Kapoian T, O'Mara NB, Singh AK, et al. Ferric gluconate reduces epoetin requirements in hemodialysis patients with elevated ferritin. *J Am Soc Nephrol* 2008;19:372-379.

71. Mandreoli M, Finelli C, Lopez A, et al. Successful resumption of epoetin alfa after rituxamab treatment in a patient with pure red cell aplasia. *Am J Kidney Dis* 2004;44(4):757-761.

72. Bennett CL, Cournoyer D, Carson KR, et al. Long-term outcome of individuals with pure red cell aplasia and antierythropoietin antibodies in patients treated with recombinant epoetin: a follow-up report from the Research on Adverse Drug Events and Reports (RADAR) Project. *Blood* 2005;106(10):3343-3347.

73. Attallah N, Osman-Malik Y, Frinak S, et al. Effect of intravenous ascorbic acid in hemodialysis patients with EPO-hyporesponsive anemia and hyperferritinemia. *Am J Kidney Dis* 2006;47(4):644-654.

74. Chan D, Irish A, Dogra G. Efficacy and safety of oral versus intravenous ascorbic acid for anaemia in haemodialysis patients. *Nephrology* 2005;10(4):336-340.

75. Gastaldello K, Vereerstraeten A, Nzame-Nze T, et al. Resistance to erythropoietin in iron-overloaded haemodialysis patients can be overcome by ascorbic acid administration. *Nephrol Dial Transplant* 1995;10(suppl 6):44-47.

76. Keven K, Kutlay S, Nergizoglu G, et al. Randomized, crossover study of the effect of vitamin C on EPO response in hemodialysis patients. *Am J Kidney Dis* 2003;41(6):1233-1239.

77. Lin CL, Hsu PY, Yang HY, et al. Low dose intravenous ascorbic acid for erythropoietin-hyporesponsive anemia in diabetic hemodialysis patients with iron overload. *Renal Failure* 2003;25(3):445-453.

78. Taji Y, Morimoto T, Okada K, et al. Effects of intravenous ascorbic acid on erythropoiesis and quality of life in unselected hemodialysis patients. *J Nephrol* 2004;17(4):537-543.

79. Tarng DC, Huang TP. A parallel, comparative study of intravenous iron versus intravenous ascorbic acid for erythropoietin-hyporesponsive anaemia in haemodialysis patients with iron overload. *Nephrol Dial Transplant* 1998;13(11)2867-2872.

80. Tarng DC, Hung SC, Huang TP. Effect of intravenous ascorbic acid medication on serum levels of soluble transferrin receptor in hemodialysis patients. *J Am Soc Nephrol* 2004;15(9):2486-2493.

81. Tarng DC, Wei YH, Huang TP, et al. Intravenous ascorbic acid as an adjuvant therapy for recombinant erythropoietin in hemodialysis patients with hyperferritinemia. *Kidney Intl* 1999;55(6):2477-2486.

82. Petrarulo F, Giancaspro V. Intravenous ascorbic acid in hemodialysis patients with functional iron deficiency. *Nephrol Dial Transplant* 2000;15:1717-1718.

83. Handelman G. Vitamin C deficiency in dialysis paitents - are we perceiving the tip of an iceberg? *Nephrol Dial Transplant* 2007;22:328-331.

84. Weiss L, Tomasello S, Barna M. [Abstr] 2008 Intravenous Ascorbic Acid (IVAA) as Adjuvant Therapy of Anemia in Patients on Chronic Hemodialysis (HD) Therapy: Effects in Pediatric and Young Adults versus Adults. Pediatric Academic Societies & Asian Society for Pediatric Research Joint Meeting. Honolulu,Hawaii; May 2008.

85. Canavese C, Petrarulo M, Massarenti P, et al. Long-term, low-dose, intravenous vitamin C leads to plasma calcium oxalate supersaturation in hemodialysis patients. *Am J Kidney Dis* 2005;45(3):540-549.

86. Worcester EM, Nakagawa Y, Bushinsky DA, et al. Evidence that serum calcium oxalate supersaturation is a consequence of oxalate retention in patients with chronic renal failure. *J Clin Invest* 1986;77(6):1888-96.

87. Marangella M, Vitale C, Petrarulo M, et al. Bony content of patients with primary hyperoxaluria or oxalosis-unrelated to renal failure. *Kidney Intl* 1995;8:182-187.

88. Evans A. Dialysis-related carnitine disorder and levocarnaitine pharmacology. *Am J Kidney Dis* 2003;4(4 suppl 4):s13-26.

89. Hoppel C. The role of carnitine in normal and altered fatty metabolism. *Am J Kidney Dis* 2003;4(4 suppl 4):s4s12.

90. Arduini A, Gorbunov N, Arrigoni-Martelli E, et al. Effects of L-carnitine and its acetate and propionate esters on the moelcular dynamics of human erythrocyte membrane. *Biochem Biophys Acta* 1993;1146:229-235.

91. McDonald R. Pentoxifylline reduces injury to isolated lungs perfused with human neutrophils. *Am Rev Respir Dis* 1991;144:1347-1350.

92. Waage A, Sorenson M, Stordal B. Differential effect of oxpentifylline on tumour necrosis factor and interleukin 6 production. *Lancet* 1990;335:543.

93. Navarro JF, Mora C, García J, et al. Effects of Pentoxifylline on the hematologic status in anaemic patients with advanced renal failure. *Scand J Urol Nephrol* 1999;33:121-125.

94. Cooper A, Mikhail A, Lethbridge MW, et al. Pentoxifylline improves hemoglobin levels in patients with erythropoietin-resistant anemia in renal failure. *J Am SocNephrol* 2004;15:1877-1882.

95. Dar Santos AE, Shalansky KF, Jastrzebski JP. Management of anemia in erythropoietin-resistant hemodialysis patients. *Annal Pharmacother* 2003;37(12):1768-1773.

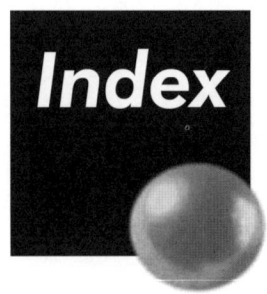

Index

*Page numbers followed by "f" denote figures; those followed by "t" denote tables.*

# A

Abscesses, 10–11
Acetaminophen
  circumcision analgesia using, 88, 91
  toxicity, 17–20
Acetylcholine receptors, 32
Acute myocardial infarction, 51–54
Adolescents, migraine headache prophylaxis in, 1
Amantadine, 27
American College of Obstetricians and Gynecologists, 64
Amitriptyline, 3–4
Androgens, 116
Anemia of chronic kidney disease
  androgens for, 116
  cardiovascular effects of, 104
  comorbid conditions that affect, 112
  erythropoiesis stimulating agents for. *See* Erythropoiesis stimulating agent(s)
  hospitalization effects on, 112
  intravenous ascorbic acid for, 114–115
  iron products for, 107–109, 113
  L-carnitine for, 115
  left ventricular hypertrophy secondary to, 104
  mortality rates, 105f
  pathophysiology of, 103
  pentoxifylline for, 115–116
  prevalence of, 103, 104f
  sequelae of, 103–104
  treatment of, 105–109
Anemia of sickle cell disease, 116
Anesthesia, for penile nerve block, 90
Angiotensin-converting enzyme inhibitors, 53, 112
Angiotensin-receptor blockers, 53, 112

Anticoagulants
  hemorrhage risks, 72
  low molecular weight heparin, 75
  warfarin. *See* Warfarin
Antiepileptic agents, 4t, 5
Apnea, 32
Arrhythmias, 32–33
Ascorbic acid, intravenous, 114–115
Aspirin-use screen, 51–54
Atrial fibrillation, 72

# B

Bactrim. *See* Cotrimoxazole
Basal insulin dosing, 39–40
Beta-blockers, 5
Bone metabolism disorder, 111
Bradycardia, 32
Brown recluse spider bite, 10f
BsmI type vitamin D receptor, 111

# C

Cancer
  prostate, 59
  soy for prevention of, 56
  "Cardio-Renal Syndrome," 104
  L-carnitine, 115
Celiac disease. *See also* Gluten
  characteristics of, 79
  clinical manifestations of, 80t
  consultation with pharmacist about, 85
  diagnosis of, 81
  gluten-free diet for, 81–82
  intestinal lesions in, 82
  management of, 81–82
  misdiagnoses, 80t
  prevalence of, 79
  vitamin deficiencies in, 82

Children's Hospital of Orange County, 98–99

Cholesterol, 55

Chronic kidney disease
anemia of. *See* Anemia of chronic kidney disease
description of, 26
pathophysiology of, 103
prevalence of, 103

Ciprofloxacin, 11

Circumcision, 87–91

Cl$_{cr}$. *See* Creatinine clearance

Clindamycin
community-associated methicillin-resistant *Staphylococcus aureus* treated with, 11
resistance to, 12–14

Clindamycin Disk Induction Test, 12–14, 13f

Coagulation factors, 71

Cockcroft-Gault equation, 23–27

Combined oral contraceptives, 64t

Community-associated methicillin-resistant *Staphylococcus aureus*, 9–11

Contraception, emergency, 63–70

Coronary heart disease, 55

Cotrimoxazole
indications for, 72
warfarin interactions with, 72–78, 73t

C-reactive protein, 111

Creatinine clearance, 23, 25, 27–28

Critical care pharmacists, 44–45, 48

Critically ill patients
glycemic control in, 43–49
hyperglycemia in, 43

CYP 2C9, 71

Cytokines, 111

**D**

"D test," 12–14, 13f

Daidzein, 56

Darbepoetin, 106

Depolarizing neuromuscular blocking agent, 31

Disk Induction Test, 12–14, 13f

Divalproex, 3, 4t, 5

Dorsal penile nerve block, 89–91

Drug(s)
erythropoiesis stimulating agent hypore sponse induced by, 112
gluten-free, 82–84

Drug dosing
adjustments in, 26–27
recommendations for, 27

Drug interactions, 72–78, 73t

Duodenal biopsy, for celiac disease, 81

**E**

Electrocardiogram, 33f

Emergency contraception, 63–70

EMLA™ cream, 88–89, 91

Epoetin alfa, 106, 107f

*erm,* 12

Erythromycin, 11

Erythropoiesis stimulating agent(s)
anemia of chronic kidney disease treated with, 106
hyporesponse to. *See* Erythropoiesis stimulating agent hyporesponse
iron evaluations in patient receiving, 108

Erythropoiesis stimulating agent hyporesponse
adjuvant therapies, 114
bone metabolism disorder as cause of, 111
L-carnitine for, 115
causes of, 108t, 108–112
cytokines and, 111
definition of, 109
drug-induced, 112
evaluation of, 112
hospitalization and, 112
infection/inflammation as cause of, 111
iron deficiency as cause of, 110, 113
pentoxifylline for, 115–116
pure red cell aplasia as cause of, 109t, 110–111, 113
treatment of, 113–116

Erythropoietin, 103, 111

17ß-Estradiol, 56

Ethinyl estradiol with levonorgestrel/norgestrel, 63

Eutectic mixture of local anesthetics (EMLA™) cream, 88–89, 91

**F**

Ferritin, 107, 113

Fluid restriction, for patent ductus arteriosus, 95

Foreskin removal. *See* Circumcision

Free fatty acid metabolism, 36–37

Functional iron deficiency, 110, 113–114

**G**

Genistein, 56

Glomerular filtration rate
calculation of, 23
Cockcroft-Gault equation, 23–25
Modification of Diet in Renal Disease, 28

Glucosuria, 35

Gluten. *See also* Celiac disease
in beauty aids, 84
definition of, 79
diet without, 81–82
in dietary supplements, 83
grains and flours that do not contain, 81t
information resources for, 84
in pharmaceutical products, 82–85

Glycemic control
in critically ill patients, 49
in intensive care unit, 43–49
mortality reductions through, 43–44
NICE-SUGAR study, 49
outpatient therapy and, 41

Gums, 83

**H**

Headaches. *See* Migraine headaches

Hemoglobin, 108

Hemoglobinopathies, 112

Hemorrhage
intracerebral, 72
intraventricular, 100

Heparin, low molecular weight, 75

High-density lipoprotein cholesterol, 55

Hospital-associated methicillin-resistant *Staphylococcus aureus,* 11

Hospitalization
anemia of chronic kidney disease affected by, 112
erythropoiesis stimulating agent hyporesponse and, 112

hyperglycemia risks, 35–41

Hyperglycemia, 35–41

Hyperkalemia, 32–34

Hypoglycemia in intensive care unit, 45, 47

Hyporesponse to erythropoiesis stimulating agents. *see* Erythropoiesis stimulating agent hyporesponse

**I**

Ibuprofen/ibuprofen lysine, 95–102

Ideal body weight, 24

Increased intracranial pressure, 32

Indomethacin, 95, 96t–97t

Infection, 111

Inflammation, 111

Insulin
hypoglycemia risks, 47
intensive vs. conventional treatment, for hyperglycemia, 43–44
sliding scale, 35–41

Intensive care unit
glycemic control in, 43–49
hypoglycemia in, 45, 47

intensive insulin treatment in, 45

Interleukin-1, 111

Interleukin-6, 111

International Classification of Headache Disorders, 2t

International Normalized Ratio, 71, 74

Intracerebral hemorrhage, 72

Intravenous ascorbic acid, 114–115

Intraventricular hemorrhage, 100

Iron deficiency, 110, 113

Iron deficiency anemia, 82

Iron products, 107–109, 113
ISIS-2 trial, 52
Isoflavones, 56–57
Isotope dilution mass spectrometry, 23

**K**

Kaplan–Meier curves, 44f
Kidney Disease Outcomes Disease Initiative, 23

**L**

Left ventricular hypertrophy, 104
Leuven II, 44–49
Levonorgestrel. *See* Plan B
Lidocaine, liposomal, 89
Liposomal lidocaine, 89
L-M-Xtrademark4 Cream, 89, 91
Local anesthesia, for penile nerve block, 90
Low molecular weight heparin, 75
Low-density lipoprotein cholesterol, 55

**M**

Magnesium supplementation, 5–6
Malignant hyperthermia, 32
Malnutrition-inflammation complex syndrome, 111
MDRD equation. *See* Modification of Diet in Renal Disease equation
Methemoglobinemia, 88
Methicillin-resistant *Staphylococcus aureus,* 9–10
Migraine headaches
    diagnostic criteria for, 2t
    incidence of, 1
    during pregnancy, 6
    prophylaxis, 2–6
    treatment of, 3–6
    triggers for, 3
$MLS_bC$, 12
$MLS_bi$, 12
Modification of Diet in Renal Disease equation
    abbreviated, 25–26
        Cockcroft-Gault equation vs., 26–27
        development of, 23, 25–26
        limitations of, 26

versions of, 26
Mogan procedure, 90
Myocardial infarction, acute, 51–54

**N**

N-acetylcysteine, 17–20
N-acetyl-L-cysteine, 18
N-acetyl-p-benzoquinoneimine, 18
National Kidney Disease Education Program, 23, 27
National Kidney Foundation, 23
National Kidney Foundation-Kidney Disease Quality Outcomes Initiative, 107–110, 114–115
Neonates
    circumcision in, 87–91
    premature, 95, 100
Neuroglycopenia, 47
Neuromuscular blocking agents, 31–34
NICE-SUGAR study, 49
Nonsteroidal anti-inflammatory drugs, 95–96, 99

**O**

Oxalosis, 115

**P**

Parathyroid hormone, 111
Patent ductus arteriosus
    Children's Hospital of Orange County study, 98–99
    definition of, 95
    fluid restriction for, 95
    ibuprofen for, 95–102
    treatment of, 95–98
Penicillin receptor binding protein 2a, 11
Penile nerve block, 89–91
Pentoxifylline, 115–116
Performance Improvement Department in hospitals, 52
Pharmaceutical products, gluten in, 82–85
Phytoestrogens, 56
Plan B®, 63–70

Postprandial glucose, 41
Pregnancy
    migraine headaches during, 6
    unintended, 63
Premature neonates, 95, 100
Prilocaine, 88
Propranolol, 3, 5
Prostaglandin E2, 96
Prostate cancer, 59
Pure red cell aplasia, 109t, 110–111, 113

## R

RABBIT 2 Trial, 39–41
Renal function calculations, 23–27
Riboflavin, 6
Ring block, 90–91
R-warfarin, 71

## S

Screenings, aspirin-use, 51–54
Sepsis, 49
Septra. *See* Cotrimoxazole
Serum creatinine, 26, 28
Sickle cell anemia, 116
Siersbaek-Nielsen Nomogram, 24
Skin abscesses, 10–11
Sliding scale insulin, 35–41
Soy, 55–61
Spider bites, 9–10
Stress-related hyperglycemia, 41
Subcutaneous ring block, 90–91
Succinylcholine, 31–34
Sucrose pacifier, 89–91
Sulfamethoxazole/trimethoprim, 11. *See also*
    Cotrimoxazole
S-warfarin, 71

## T

Testosterone, 56–59, 58t
Thromboembolism, 77
Topiramate, 4t, 5
Transferrin, 107

Transient hypoglycemia, 47
Tricyclic antidepressants, 3–4
Tumor necrosis factor alpha, 111

## U

Unintended pregnancies, 63
Urine, creatine excretion in, 24

## V

Verapamil, 5–6
Vitamin D receptor, 111
Vitamin deficiencies, 82
Vitamin K, 71, 73t
Vitamin K epoxide reductase complex 1, 71

## W

Warfarin
    atrial fibrillation treated with, 72
    cotrimoxazole interactions with, 72–78, 73t
    drug interactions, 72–78, 73t
    factors that affect, 71
    indications for, 71
    International Normalized Ratio for, 71, 74
Weight gain, 3–4
World Health Organization, 66

## Y

Yuzpe regimen, 63